HOLLYWOOD LEGS

PAT HENRY

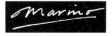

ABOUT THE AUTHOR

Pat Henry, MIHCA, AABS, yoga therapist, has lectured on yoga and health throughout the USA and Europe. His appearances on RTE television reached an audience of over 6 million people in Ireland and England over a three-month period. He has participated in radio programmes, and his articles on fitness have appeared in leading newspapers and magazines. As a personal trainer he has worked with many of the top stars. Among his clients have been Jeananne Crowley, Ellen Barkin, Gabriel Byrne, Matt Dillon, Julia Ormond, Joanne Whalley-Kilmer, Angeline Ball, Johnny Logan, Dolores O'Riordan, Adèle King (Twink), Fionnuala Sherry, David Bowie, Michael Flatley, Jean Butler, Wayne Sleep – to mention but a few . . .

His fitness centre in Dublin, which he established in 1986, is open to men and women of all ages.

First published in 1997 by
Marino Books
An imprint of Mercier Press
16 Hume Street Dublin 2

Trade enquiries to CMD Distribution
55A Spruce Park Stillorgan Industrial
Estate Blackrock County Dublin

© Pat Henry 1997

ISBN 1 86023 056 3

10 9 8 7 6 5 4 3 2 1

A CIP record for this title is available
from the British Library

Cover and inside photographs by
Vincent O'Byrne
Models Karen O'Reilly (leg exercises)
and Lesley Robertson (stretches)
Cover design by Penhouse Design
Set by Richard Parfrey
Printed in Ireland by ColourBooks,
Baldoyle Industrial Estate, Dublin 13

DEDICATION

Dedicated to Marie and our sons Cathal and Karl. Without Marie there would be no book or gym. In gratitude for her great support, encouragement and faith when I had none, and for her tireless energy and love. Also to happy memories of my mother and father, who would have loved to see this book and to Marie's mother and her late father.

ACKNOWLEDGEMENTS

A special thanks to all who helped to put this book together. To Jeananne Crowley for the call. To Lesley Robertson, manageress at our Dublin centre, who put together exercises and photos. To Michael Cantwell, dietician and masseur *extraordinaire* for assembling our diet programme and menus. To Vincent O'Byrne, master photographer and artist, for the photographs. To Sean Nolan and Sean Lawlor for all their help and encouragement. To Bill Cunningham, a great trainer. To John Synott for having faith in the unknown. To Chris Roche, sparring partner, walking buddy and great publicist. To Adrian Copeland for the £150 and the encouragement. To Billy Parker for the guitar lessons. To Austin Kenny for your lessons in diplomacy. To all of you, I truly value your friendship.

CONTENTS

INTRODUCTION

Over the past twenty-five years I have worked with thousands of women of all shapes and sizes. The main areas of concern have been the legs and the bottom, and I have found that the correct exercises combined with an improved eating plan will always yield results. I am not suggesting that when you finish you will have legs like Cindy Crawford or Naomi Campbell. They were given by the man or woman above. Genetics play a huge part in body shape but you *can* improve on whatever you have. You may have exercised before but seen little improvement. This may have been the result of incorrect exercise. For example, high-impact aerobics, constant pounding on the step or floor or any hard surface will, I believe, widen the hips and increase the size of your thighs and calves. Your body will always try to protect you from damage and injury by increasing the level of fat. When the body is under attack it will shut down the fat-burning process to restore energy. As is the case with crash diets, your main loss would be of muscle, not fat, so you could even end up softer than you were at the beginning.

1

THE EXERCISE PROGRAMME

MOTIVATION

If you are aiming to reduce fat in one area, forget it. Your body-fat composition will reduce all over when you change your diet. The time spent exercising should be no more than a maximum of one hour three times a week or five times a week when you progress a little further. Choose a time when you are on your own or with friends who are on a similar programme. This will encourage you to keep working out. The most suitable time for exercise depends on your energy levels. Some people prefer early morning. This is really the best time for your work-out as it will improve your circulation and speed up your metabolism. It will also get your engine warmed up to help make you feel sharper during the day. But you should pick your own time – this is your quality time for yourself – and make a commitment for six weeks. Stick to the programme, keep a note of how you feel and how your daily eating plan is going. This will help you to become more focused on what you want to achieve.

It might be a good idea when embarking on an adventure like this to make it top secret, for your eyes only. If you tell people of your plan they may say, 'Here she goes again – it will never work.' Remarks like this may not be meant seriously but you may take them seriously and that could be the end of your plan. Only tell those who are really behind you.

The exercises you will be doing have been developed over years and I have found this combination to be the most effective for all ages. There is no need to overload and be so sore that you can hardly walk the next day. Burn and pain are not necessary. I call this programme cosmetic exercising because it aims to give a nicer shape and the illusion of length rather than shorten the look of the thighs by wrong exercises.

BODY TYPES

Before you start on a leg-improving programme let's look at the design of the programme, which takes into consideration the fact that there are different body types; endomorph, mesomorph and ectomorph. You may fit into one of the types or, more likely, be a combination of two or more types. If you are, for example, the mesomorph type, strong, heavy-boned with wide hips and heavy-set legs, you will never end up looking like Twiggy but you can make a great improvement. Some typical frame combinations are:

- The typical tomboy look – lean features, broad shoulders, small waist and normally small joints.
- The pear shape – soft muscle tone, large tummy, holds on to the fat in the lower region, the hips and thighs.
- The rounder shape – overweight, large-breasted, large tummy and arms and a very soft look to the body.

Whatever your type, you will see great improvement once you change your diet, exercise three times a week and supplement the exercise with brisk walking, swimming, weight-training or any sport that enhances your figure and improves your energy and self-esteem.

ENDOMORPH   MESOMORPH   ECTOMORPH

The main muscle groups we will be working are:

1   The *quadricepses* (quads): the muscles at the front of the thighs. The quads are the main shaper of the front of the thighs. Their other functions include giving the power to run and kick.

2   The *hamstrings*: the muscles at the back of the thighs. This is a three-part muscle group that works the hip and the buttocks. In order to create balance, the hamstrings should be worked in combination with the front thigh. Some people ignore this but the result can be a very unsymmetrical look to the legs.

3   The *glutei* (glutes): the bottom area. The exercises we will be doing will help to firm and tighten up your bottom and to lift it as well.

4   The *abductors*: the muscles on the outside of the thighs and hips. This is one of the problem areas but when the correct exercises are followed it can be worked very effectively.

5   The *adductors*: the inside thigh muscles. This area is generally soft and sometimes hard to work but when firm, the muscles can give a nice balanced look, especially from the front view.

6   The *calves*: the lower legs. Exercising the calves can help to give the legs symmetry. Women who wear very high-heeled shoes sometimes develop the calf very high up. This gives a bulky look at the back of the knee. When you are finished your day's work try to follow our stretch routine for the lower calves given in this book. This will help to lengthen the calf muscles and give that diamond look to your calves.

HOW TO BENEFIT
FROM THE PROGRAMME

Before you start the programme make sure you have no medical problems, back problems or hip soreness. If you feel you may have, consult your GP. If you feel unwell at any stage, stop immediately. Look out for signs of stress like breathlessness or feeling dizzy. Allow at least an hour-and-a-half after food before beginning your routine. Work at your own pace. Don't push yourself too hard. Just do one set of exercises (the number of repetitions is given with each exercise) on each of three days for the first week. The second week you can move up to two sets and on the third week do three sets. If you can handle this work with ease, start to exercise five times a week, making sure not to strain your lower back or your legs.

It may take a little longer than this to reach three sets five days a week but do it in your own time. Your maximum exercise time should be one hour, allowing time for stretching and cooling down/relaxing. Examples of stretching exercises and advice on relaxation and massage are given in this book. When you reach five times weekly you will definitely see improvements *if* you have also been following your diet plan. Remember that the real purpose of exercise is to increase your energy, improve your metabolism, tone up slack muscles and provide a feeling of wellbeing.

Devoting three to five hours a week to yourself is not much. This should be your quality time. You deserve this for the new you.

I can honestly say that the exercise programme you are about to start has produced the best results for women of all ages from sixteen to seventy. Combined with a low-fat eating plan and a better mental image of what you want to achieve, this programme will definitely optimise your figure.

STRETCHES

These stretches should be done at the beginning and the end of the exercise routine. Each stretch should be held for a count of 10 and repeated 5 times.

COBRA (1)

Lie on tummy, hands either side of shoulder for gentle support.

COBRA (2)

Rise up using back and keeping hips pressed to floor, then bring head to fully upright position.
Working: lower back, spine and neck

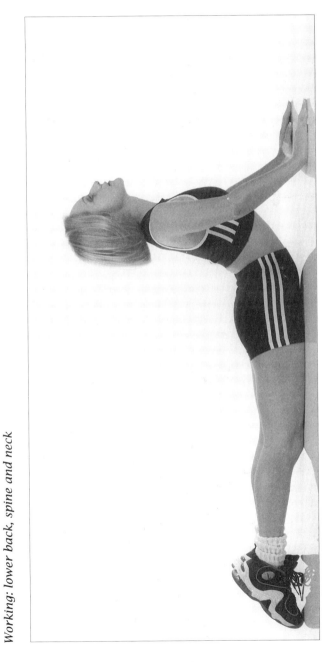

HAMSTRING STRETCH (1)

Lie on back, knees bent, back firmly on floor.

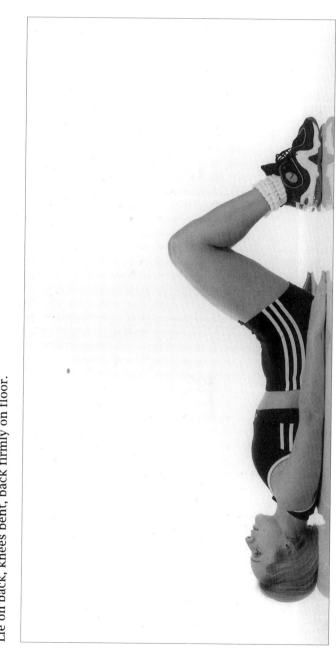

HAMSTRING STRETCH (2)

Bend one leg and raise other leg. Holding leg above or below knee joint, gently stretch back. Return foot to floor.

Working: hamstring.

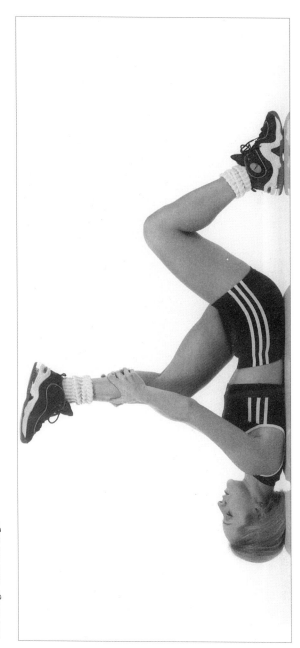

HIP STRETCH (1)

Lying on back, cross one leg over supporting leg.

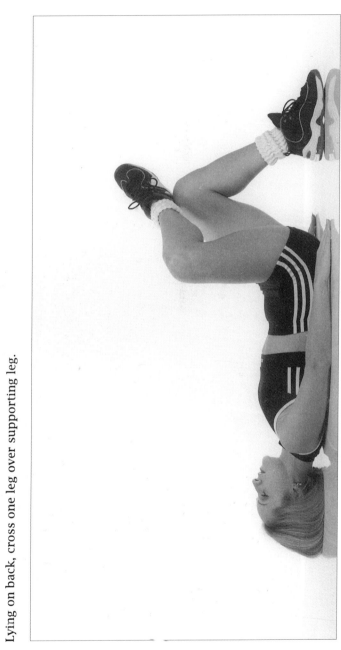

HIP STRETCH (2)

Bring legs towards chest, holding thigh to increase stretch. Slowly lower.

Working: hip and bottom.

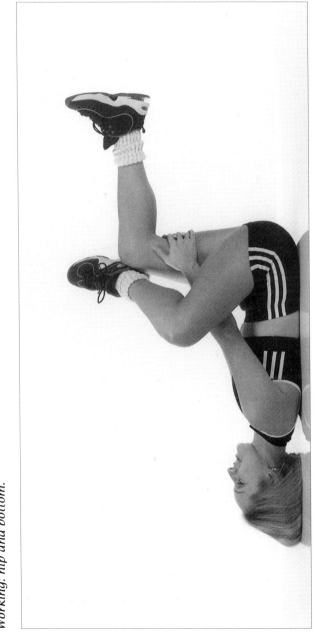

SIDE STRETCH (1)

Standing with feet wider than hip-width apart, bend knees softly.

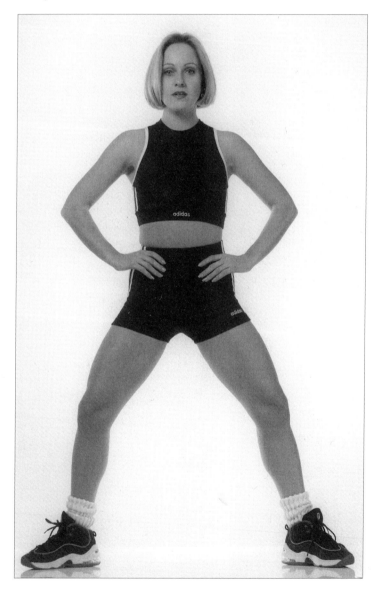

SIDE STRETCH (2)

Lean on one leg, supporting lower back, and stretch other arm out, stretching side.

Working: side and waist.

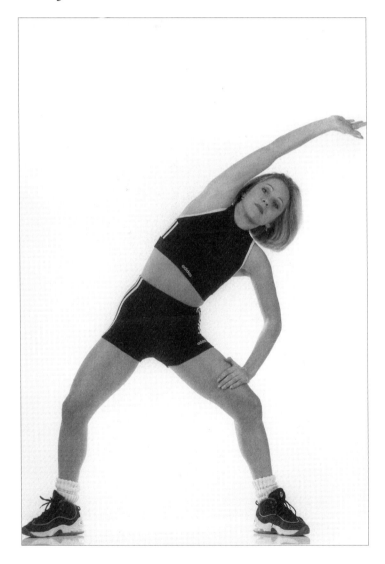

QUAD STRETCH

Standing on both feet, holding support, bend one knee. Hold bent leg at ankle, keeping knees together. Gently stretch quad and slightly bend supporting leg.

Working: quadriceps (front of thighs).

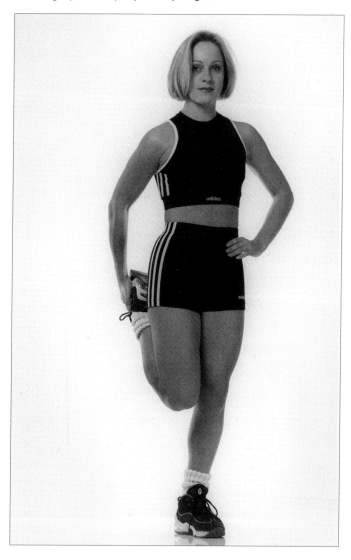

TWENTY-FIVE EXERCISES
FOR THE LEGS

1

SQUATS (1)

Start with feet further than hip-width apart, toes and knees turned outwards.

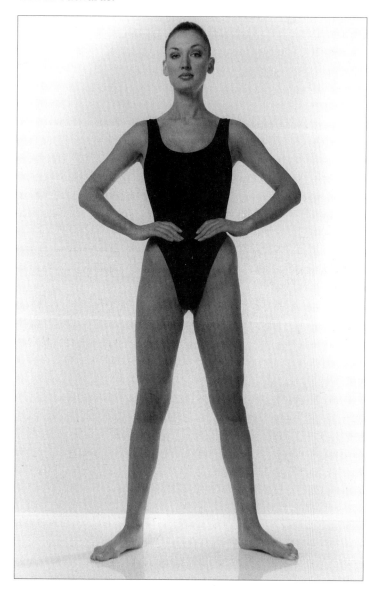

SQUATS (2)

Bend knees, keeping feet flat. Do not allow knees over toes.
Keep tummy pulled in and back straight.
20 reps; working thighs.

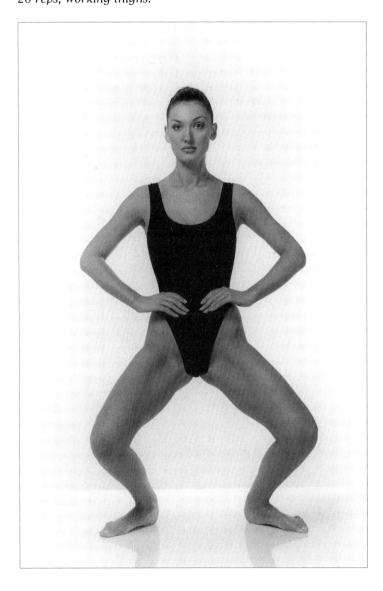

2

SQUAT KICKS (1)

As with previous exercise, start with feet apart, hands on hips.

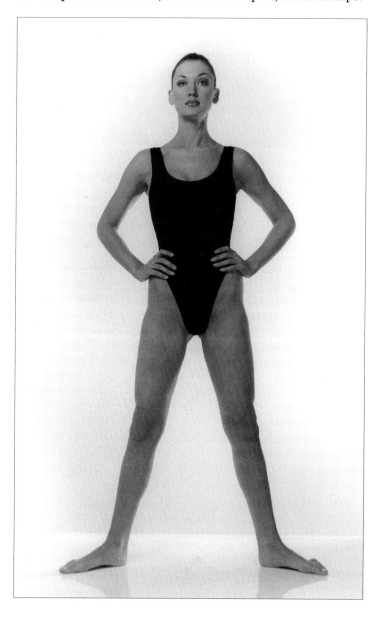

SQUAT KICKS (2)

Lower body into squat.

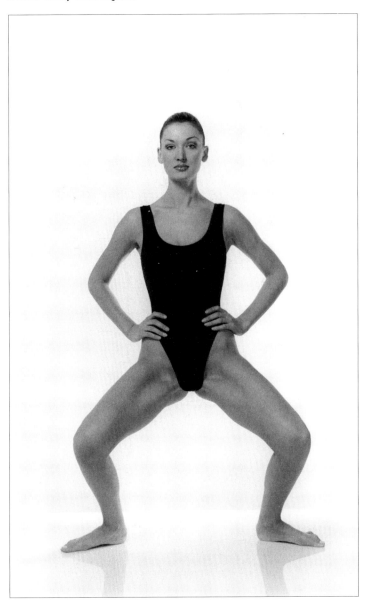

SQUAT KICKS (3)

Straighten one leg while kicking other leg upwards. Return to original starting position.

Repeat each side, 20 reps altogether; working thighs.

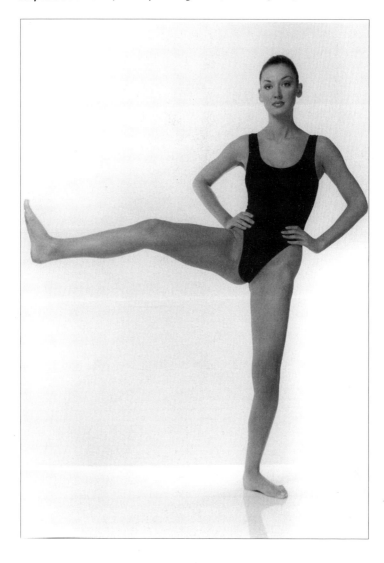

3

3-WAY SQUAT A (1)

Raise heels four inches, toes pointing forward, arms folded.

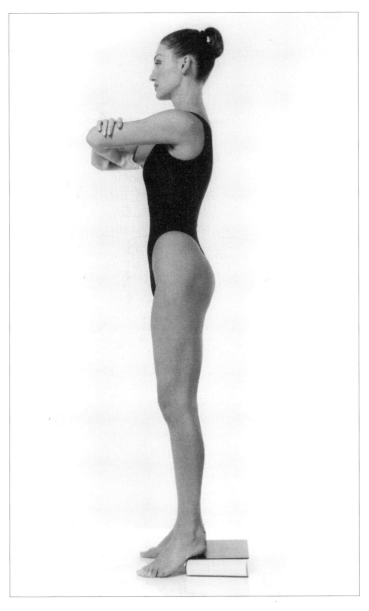

3-WAY SQUAT A (2)
Bend knees, sliding body forward and keeping knees, hips and shoulders in line. At lowest position the shoulders are over the heels. Slide back to starting position.

5 reps

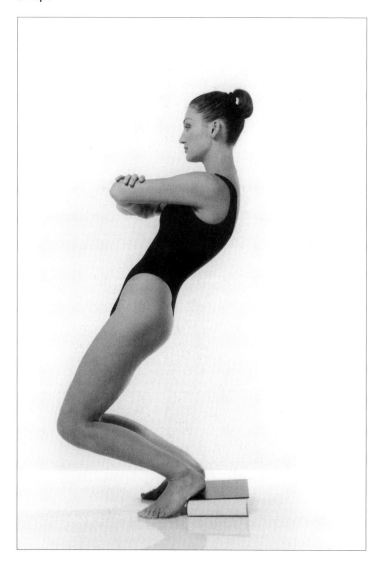

3-WAY SQUAT B (1)

Stand with heels raised.

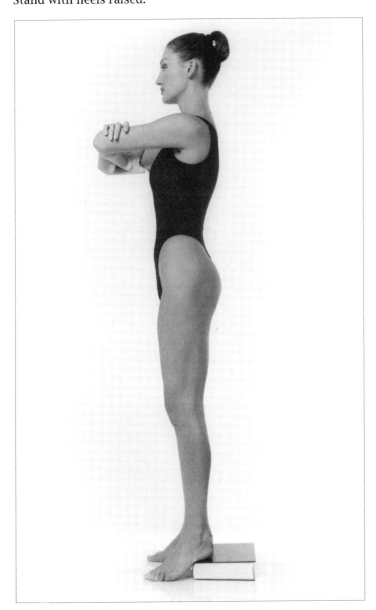

3-WAY SQUAT B (2)

Bend knees and drop hips back, sitting on heels.

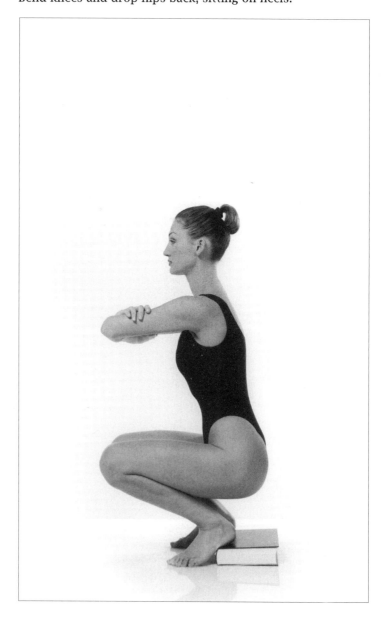

3-WAY SQUAT B (3)

Flush hips forward in one move to a flat back. Slide up to standing position in one movement.

5 reps

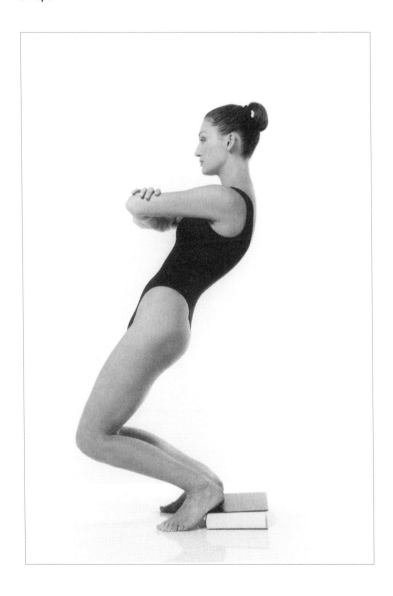

3-WAY SQUAT C (1)

Sit on heels.

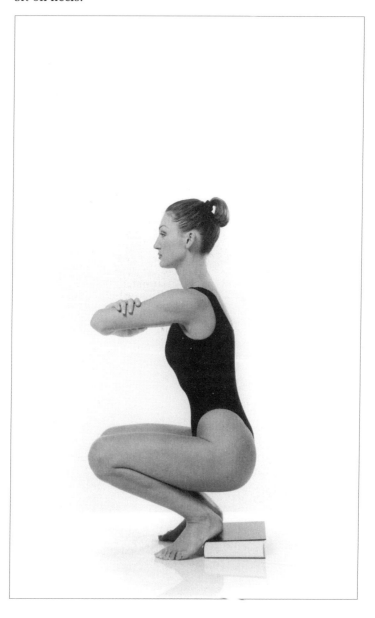

3-WAY SQUAT C (2)

Flush hips forward as B then drop back to sitting on heels.
5 reps; working front of thighs. Creates illusion of length.

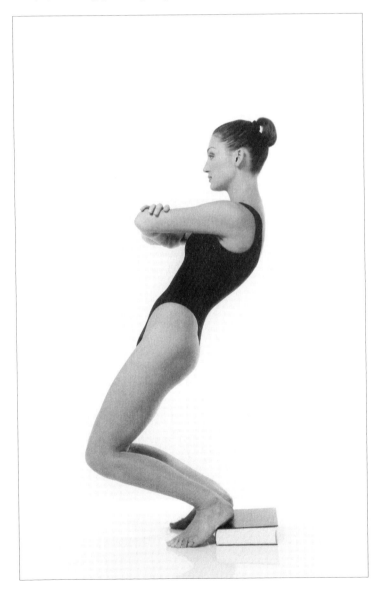

4

3-WAY PELVIC SCOOP A (1)

Standing on toes, heels together and toes turned outwards, hold bar (or chair, or wall) for support, keeping back straight. Slightly bend knees.

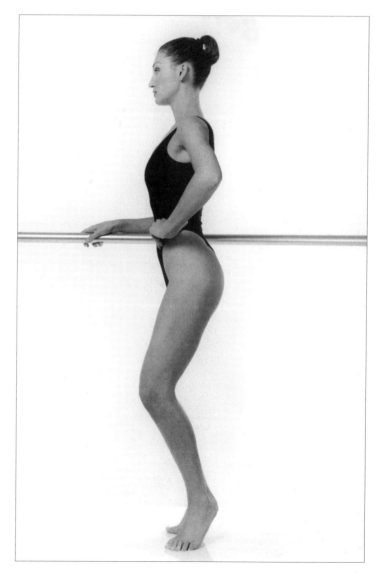

3-WAY PELVIC SCOOP A (2)

Scoop pelvis upwards and forward. Return pelvis to alignment. *Do once.*

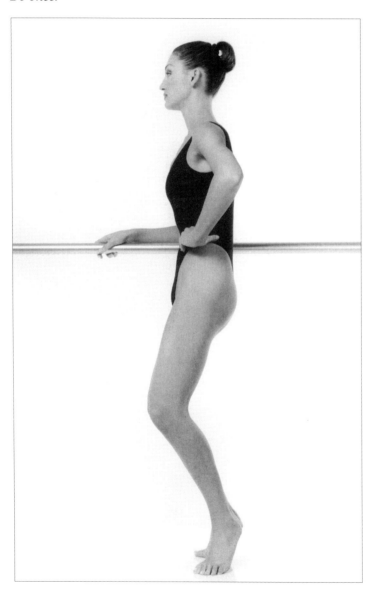

3-WAY PELVIC SCOOP B (1)
Now bending knees further, lower body a couple of inches.

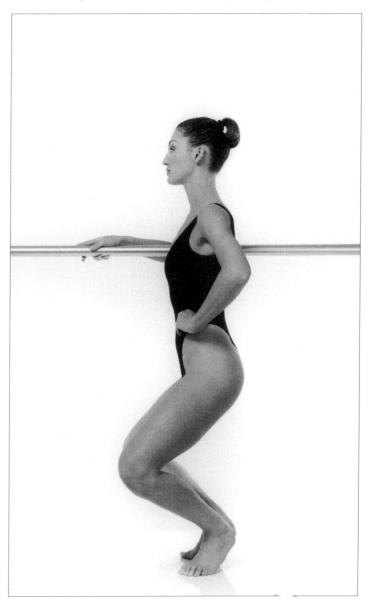

3-WAY PELVIC SCOOP B (2)

Repeat pelvic scoop. Return to correct alignment.
Do once.

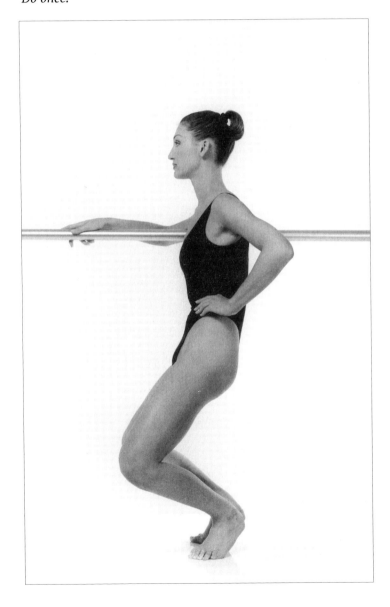

3-WAY PELVIC SCOOP C (1)

Move lower once again so body is closer to heels.

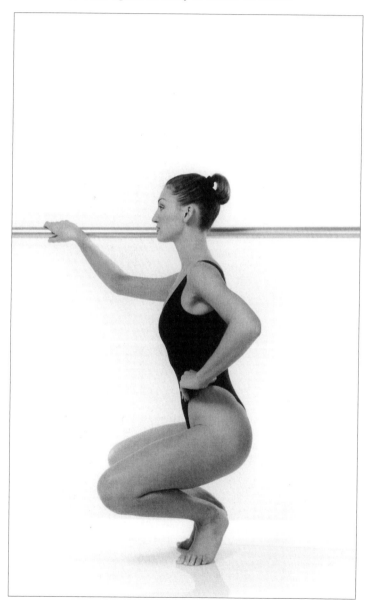

3-WAY PELVIC SCOOP C (2)

Repeat pelvic scoop. Return to correct alignment. *(Do once)*
Raising body to middle level, as in B, *repeat once.* Lastly,
returning to first level (A), *repeat once.*

*Repeat sequence 10 times; working thighs, bottom and lower
tummy.*

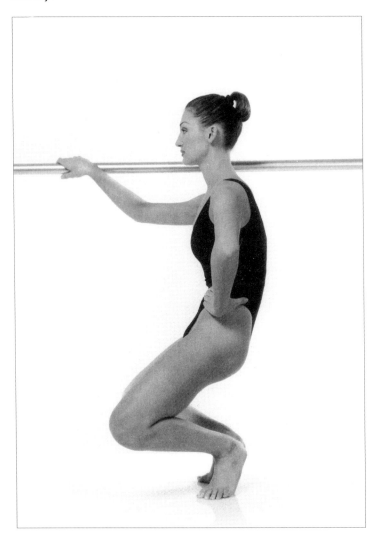

5

PLIÉ ON TOES (1)

Standing on toes, heels together, toes turned outwards, hold on to bar for support, keeping back straight.

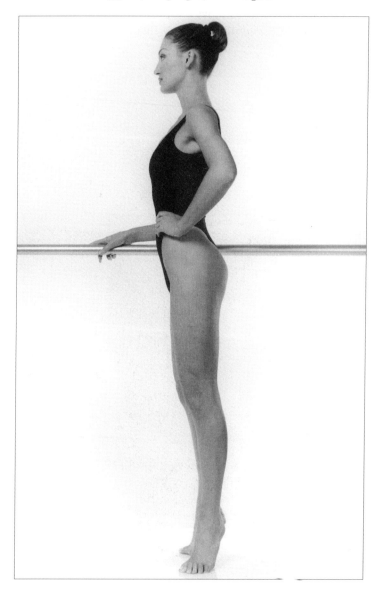

PLIÉ ON TOES (2)

Bend knees slowly, lowering body to heels. Return to original position, pulling inner thighs in. Try to keep movement continuous, not sitting in lowered position.

20 reps; working inner thighs.

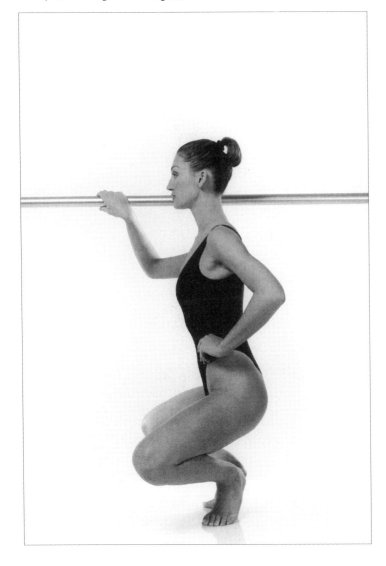

LUNGES (1)

Stand with feet together, hands on hips.

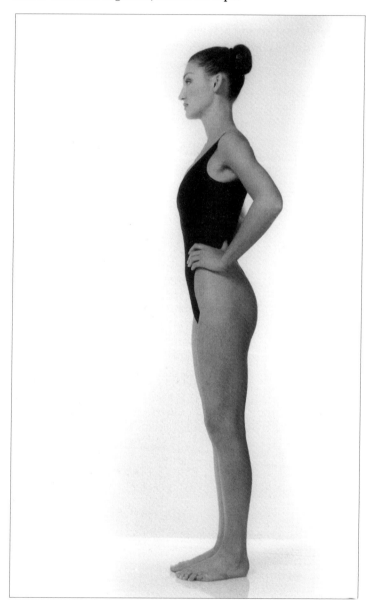

LUNGES (2)

Step out with one foot. Bring far enough in front to ensure knee is in line with ankle. Back knee bends, lowering to ground. Push off front leg back to starting position.

20 reps each leg; working front of thigh and bottom.

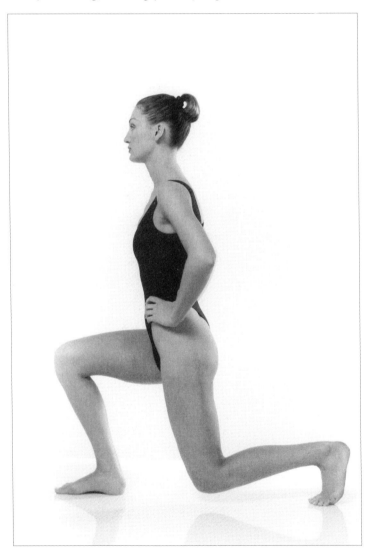

7

KNEE RAISES (1)

Stand with hands on hips; keep supporting leg soft. If necessary, support yourself on a chair or against the wall.

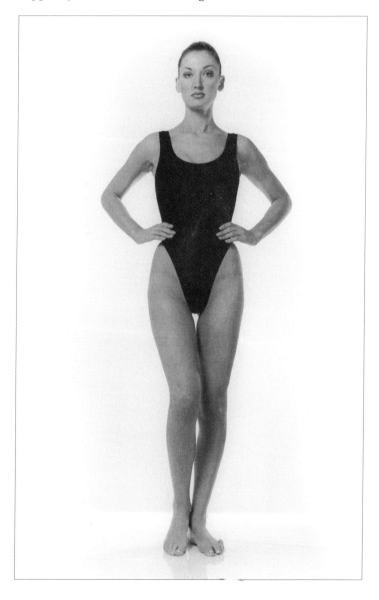

KNEE RAISES (2)

Bending knee, raise other leg to hip level. Return to ground.

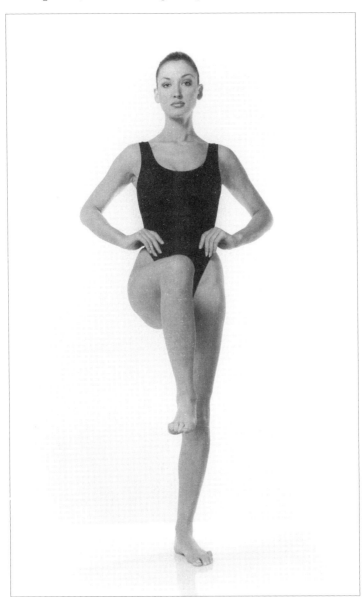

KNEE RAISES (3)

Now raise knee turned outwards, then return to start.
20 reps; working hip.

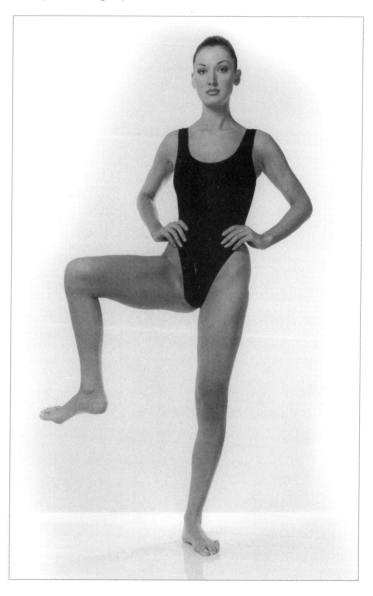

8

3-WAY LEG EXTENSION A (1)

Raise one knee to hip level. If necessary, support yourself on a chair or against the wall.

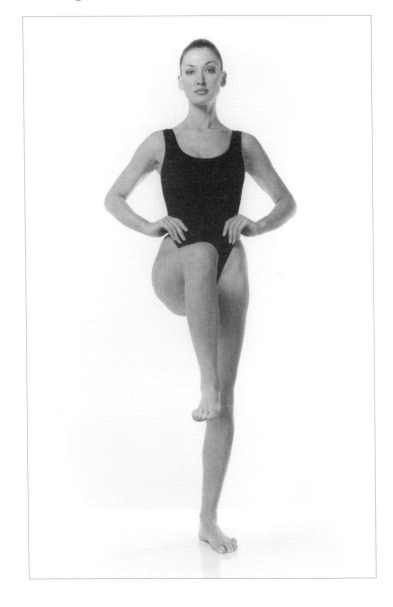

3-WAY LEG EXTENSION A (2)

Keep foot flexed, straighten leg in front and return.
20 reps; working front of thigh.

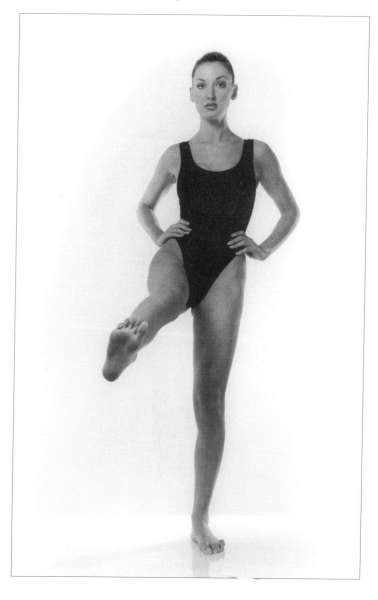

3-WAY LEG EXTENSION B

Keeping knee in same position, turn lower leg outwards. Bring heel back towards bottom, then straighten leg.

20 reps; working outer thigh.

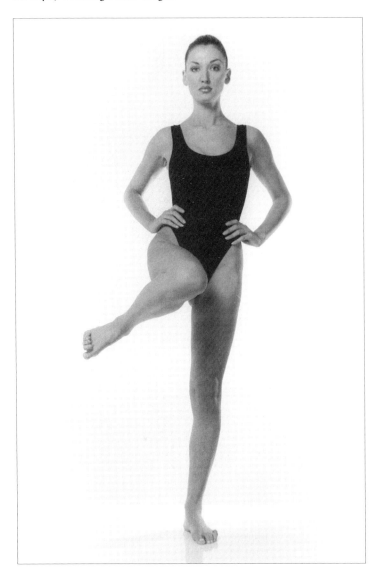

3-WAY LEG EXTENSION C

Keeping knee in same position, turn lower leg inwards, flexing foot over supporting leg. Straighten leg and return inwards.
20 reps; working inner thigh.

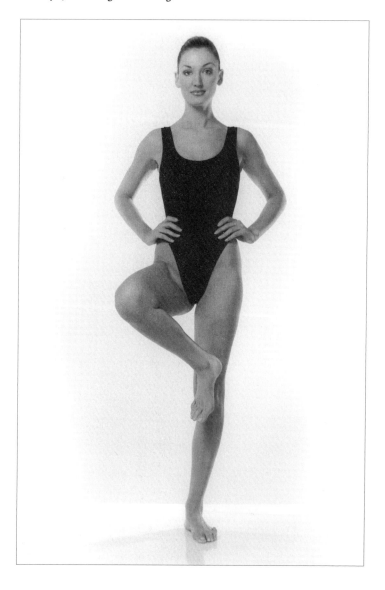

THIGH BICEP CURL (1)

Stand on both feet with hands on hips.

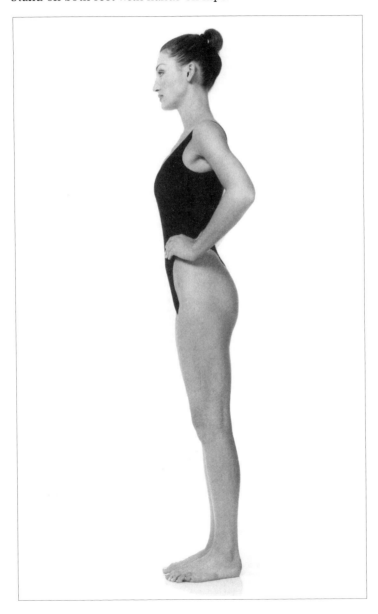

THIGH BICEP CURL (2)

Bend one leg. Bring heel in towards bottom, squeezing hamstring. Lower to ground.

20 reps; working hamstring.

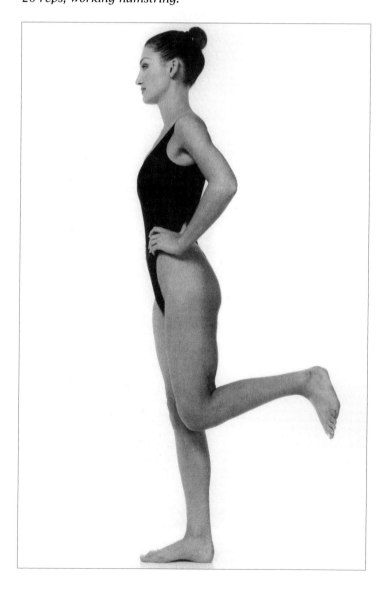

10

CALF RAISE (1)

Stand on both feet, hands on hips.

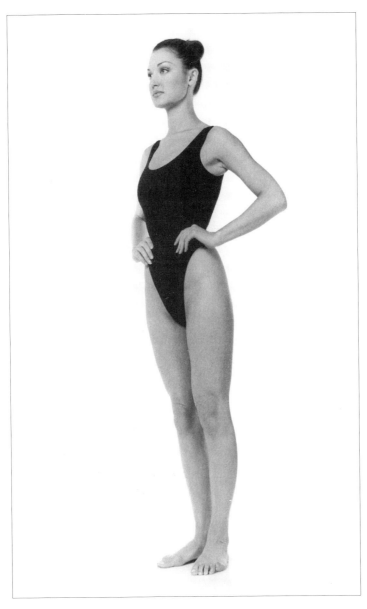

CALF RAISE (2)

Rise up on toes. Lower back to ground.

20 reps; working calves.

11

TOE TAPPING (1)

With feet slightly apart, bend knees. Lower body into sitting position. Place hands on one thigh.

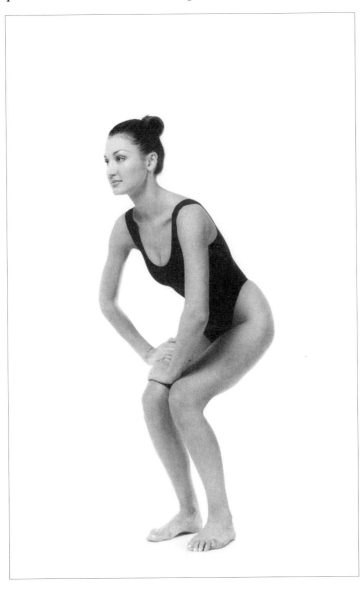

TOE TAPPING (2)

Tap toe of other leg, keeping heel on ground.

20 reps each leg; working front of lower leg.

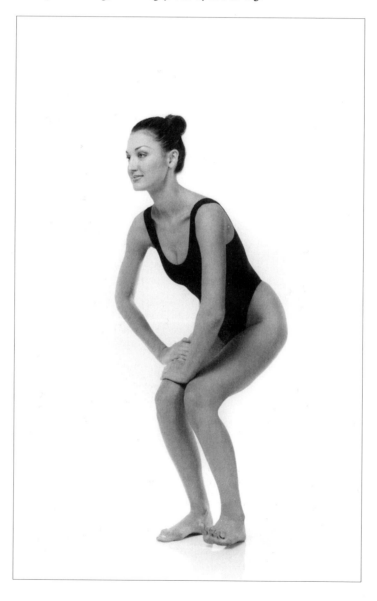

12

SIDE LEG RAISES (1)

Lying on side, bend underneath leg to give stable base. Keep hip pointing downwards, foot flexed and toe pointing down.

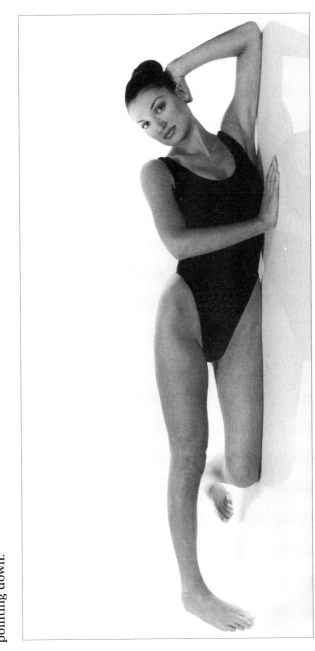

SIDE LEG RAISES (2)

Leading up with heel, raise leg and lower.

20 reps each leg; working hip and outer thigh.

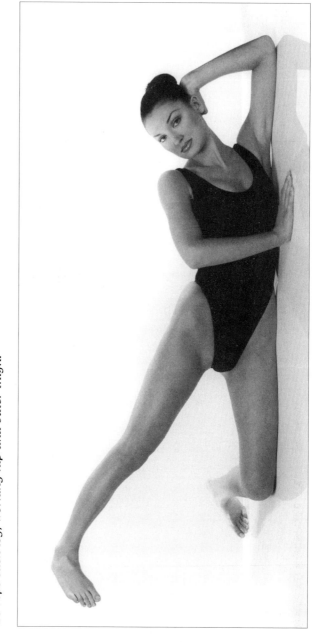

13

KNEE TO CHEST LEG EXTENSION (1)

Lying on side, bend underneath leg. Place hand in front for support. Bring knee in between chest and hand.

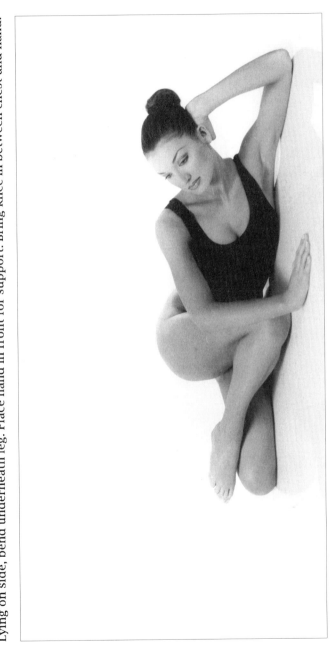

KNEE TO CHEST LEG EXTENSION (2)

Straighten leg. Lead back with heel and bring knee back in front of chest.

20 reps each leg; working hip and bottom.

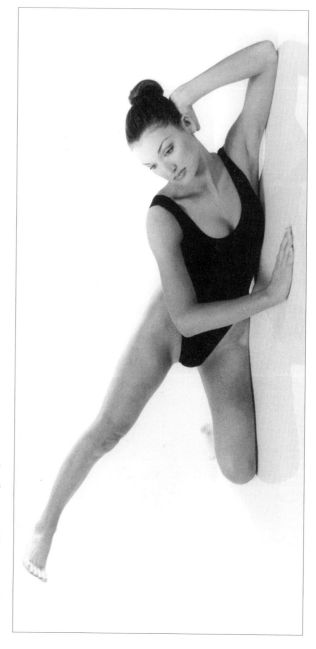

14

HIP SQUEEZE (1)

Lie on side, both legs bent and in front of body.

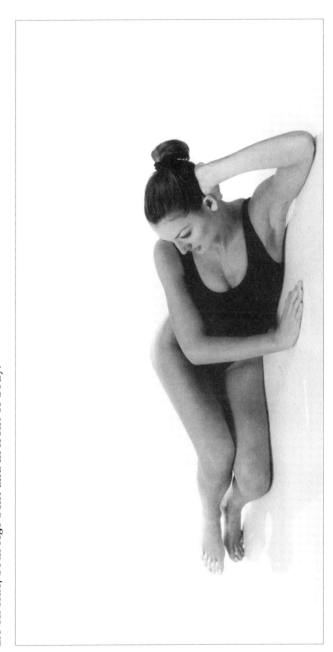

HIP SQUEEZE (2)

Raise top leg, keeping hips aligned. Return together. *Tip: don't let hip roll back. 20 reps each side; working hip.*

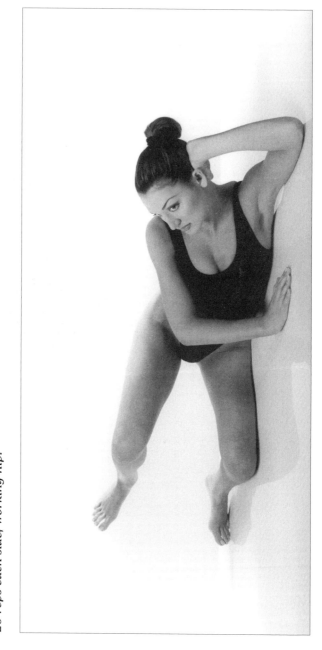

15

STRAIGHT LEG SQUEEZE (1)

As for previous exercise, lie on side, both legs bent and in front of the body. Straighten top leg.

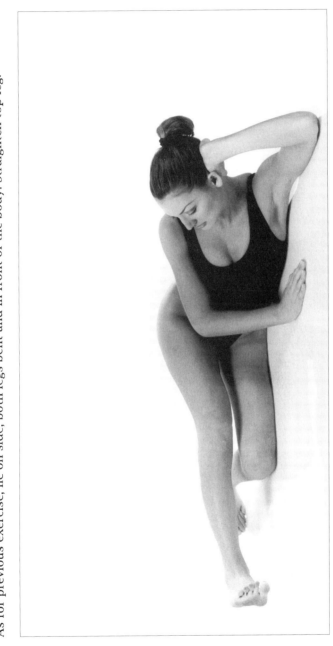

STRAIGHT LEG SQUEEZE (2)
Raise leg. A couple of inches is enough.
20 reps each side; working outer thigh and hip.

16

INNER THIGH LIFTS (1)
Lying on side, bend top knee. Lying knee on ground, straighten underneath leg.

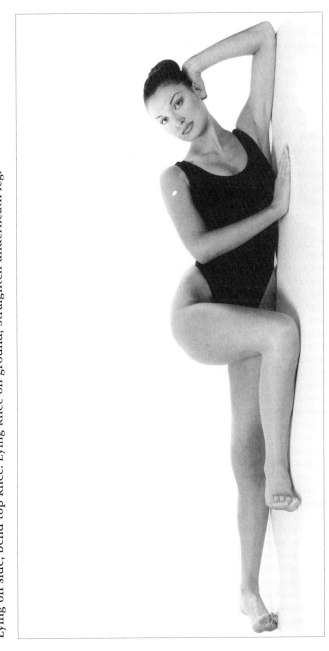

INNER THIGH LIFTS (2)

Raise leg a couple of inches, squeezing inner thigh.

20 reps each leg; working inner thigh.

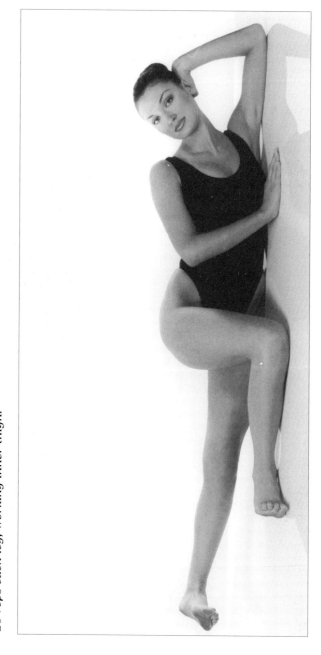

17

INNER THIGH PRESS (1)

Lying on side, bend top knee. Lower upper leg to ground. Place foot on straightened leg, adding resistance.

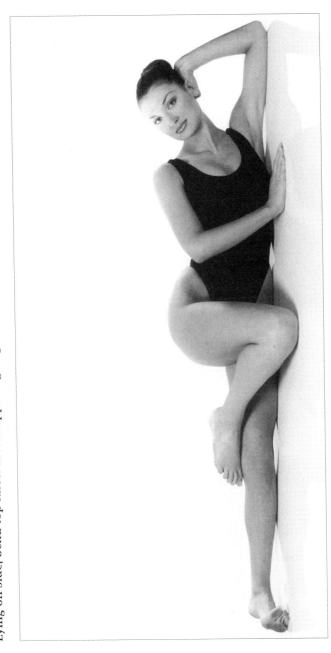

INNER THIGH PRESS (2)

Raise lower leg a couple of inches and return to floor. *Tip:* try to place foot on to thigh rather than knee joint. *20 reps each leg; working inner thigh.*

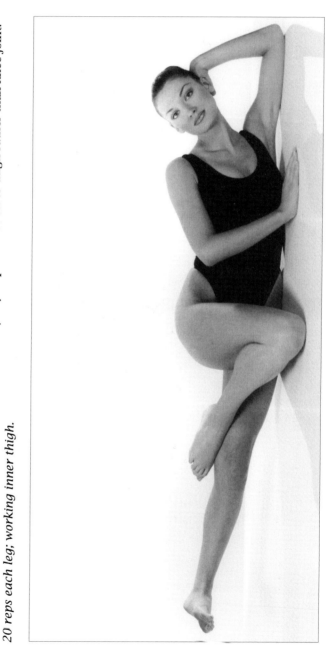

18

BOTTOM SQUEEZES

Sitting on one side, hip rolled forward, bring underneath leg in front of body for support. Raise top leg, knee bent. Bring knee back in line with hip and pulse knee back.

50 pulses each side; working bottom.

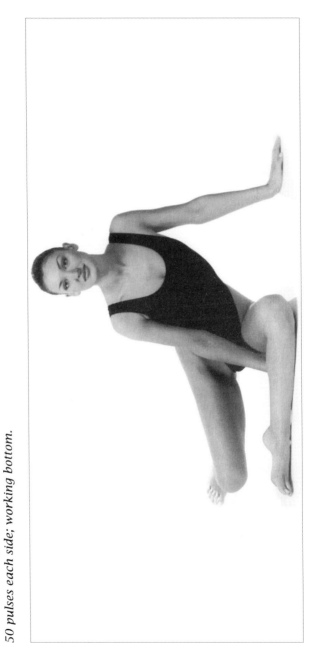

19

SITTING LEG RAISE

Sitting on one side, bend supporting leg. With hip rolled forward, straighten top leg and pulse upwards. *Tip: if you have difficulty raising, lean down on your side. Eventually you will be able to sit upright. 50 pulses each side; working outer thigh.*

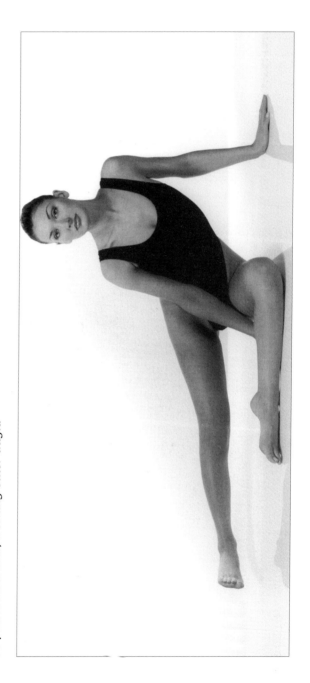

20

KNEE RAISES (1)
On all fours, raise one leg to hip level.

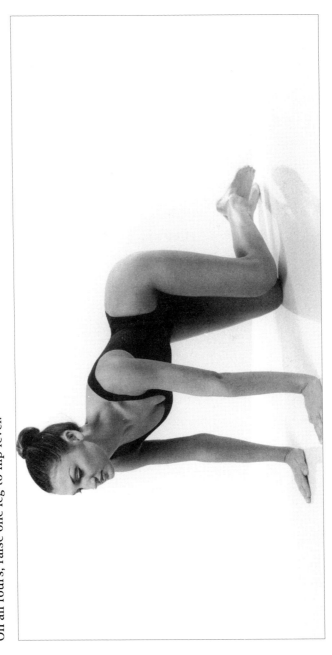

KNEE RAISES (2)

Lower back down. *Tip:* leg that is being raised should stay in line and knee should stay level with toe. Watch that the back stays in line.

20 reps each side; working hip.

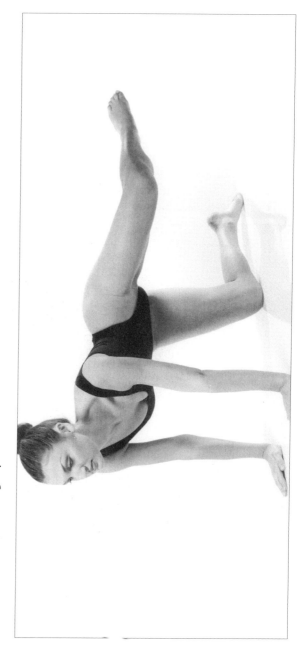

21

HAMSTRING AND BOTTOM RAISES (1)

Support upper body on elbows, with supporting knee bent. Stretch back leg out.

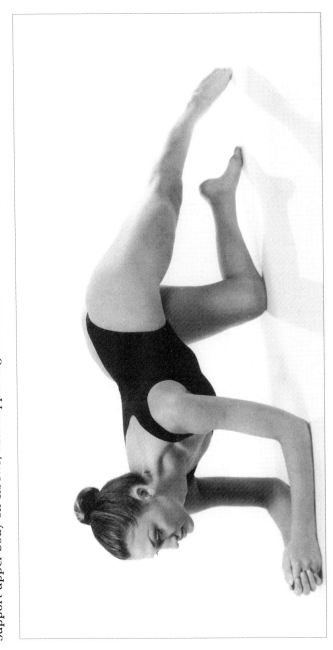

HAMSTRING AND BOTTOM RAISES (2)

Raise leg upwards with heel leading, keeping leg straight. Lower back to ground.
20 reps each leg; working hamstring and bottom.

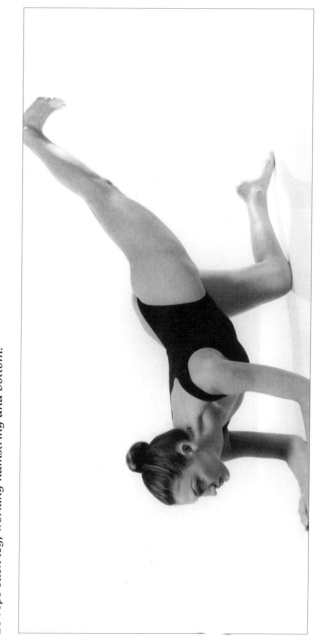

22

SCISSORS A (1)

Lie on back, hands under bottom. Both legs are raised and straight.

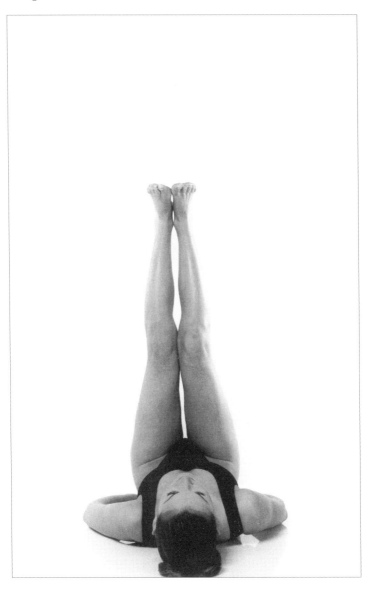

SCISSORS A (2)

Bring legs as far apart as comfortable. Bring back to centre. *20 reps; working inner thighs.*

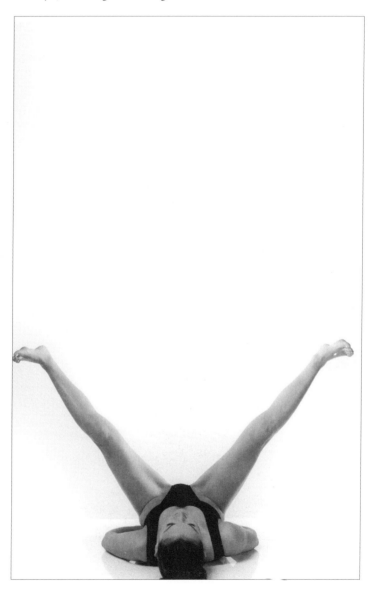

SCISSORS B

As before, separate legs. When bringing back to centre cross legs over.

20 reps; working inner thighs.

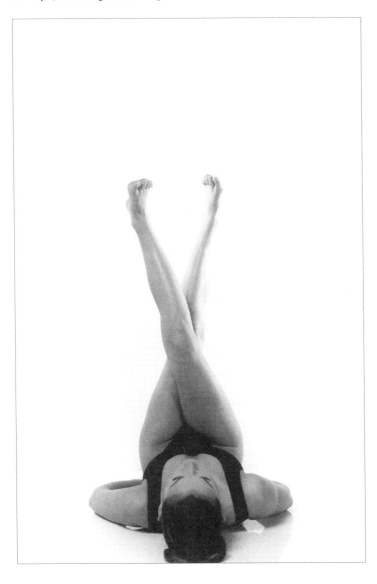

SCISSORS C

Finally, once legs are separated, squeeze in half-way and repeat.
20 reps; working inner thighs.

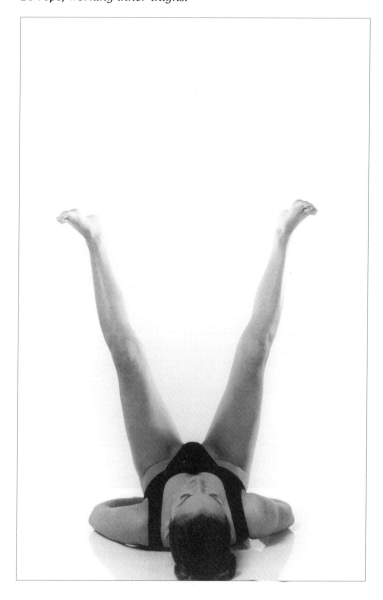

23

SCISSORS WITH PLIÉ A

Begin as for previous exercise, lying on back with hands under bottom to support lower back. Separate legs wide and bring back to centre as Scissors B.

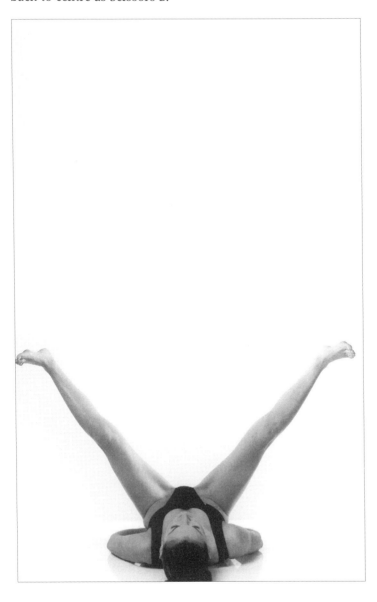

SCISSORS WITH PLIÉ B (1)

Once legs meet, bring the soles of feet together. Bend knees.

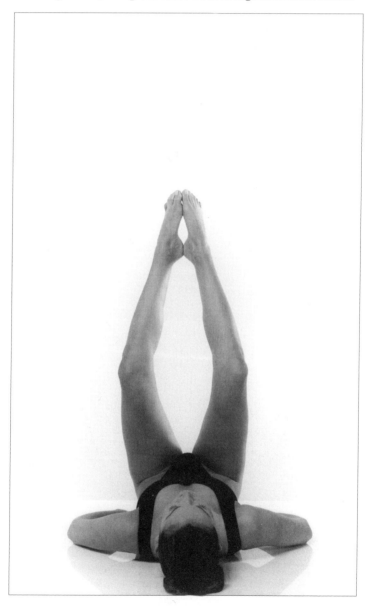

SCISSORS WITH PLIÉ B (2)

Lowering feet to body, return to straight leg.

20 reps of sequence; working inner thigh.

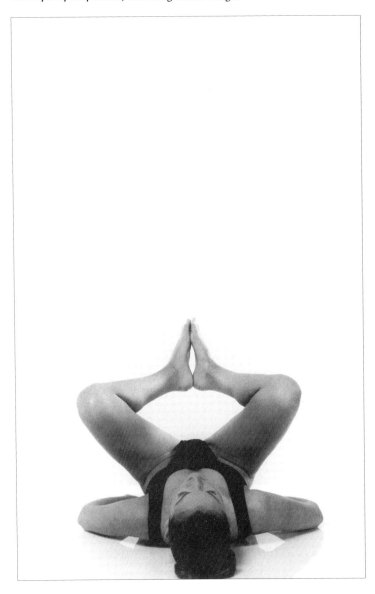

24

PELVIC SCOOP (1)

Kneel with feet flat on floor, arms raised and outstretched, with fingers linked and backs of hands facing you.

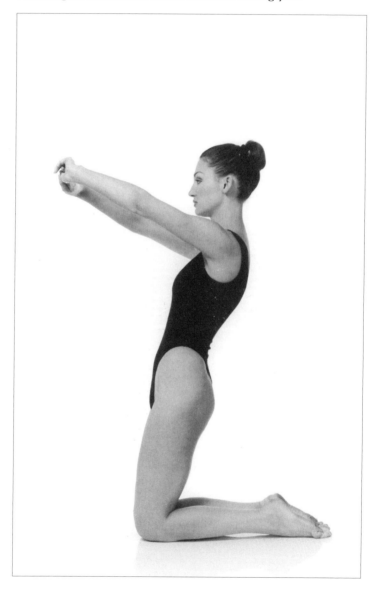

PELVIC SCOOP (2)

Lower bottom to knees, sticking bottom out and keeping back flat.

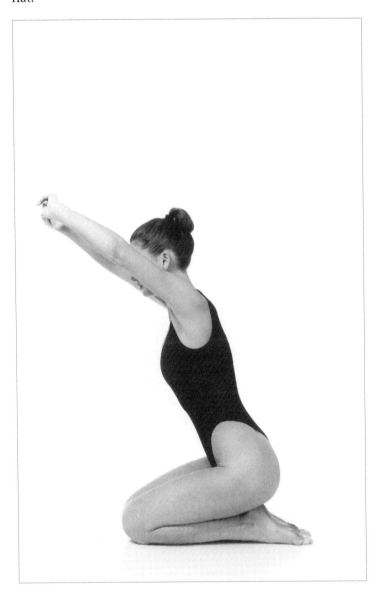

PELVIC SCOOP (3)

As bottom reaches heels, scoop hips upwards, pulling stomach in. Then rise to starting position.

20 reps; working front of thigh.

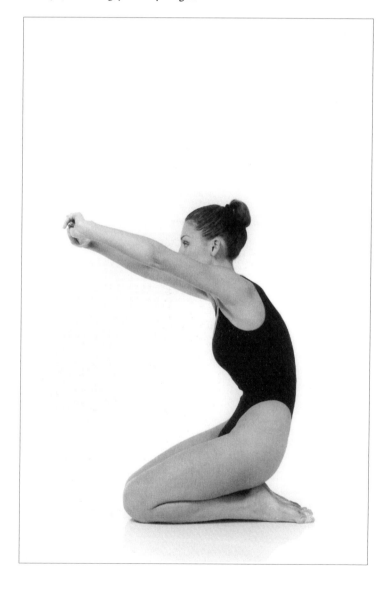

25

ARABIAN NIGHTS A (1)

Sitting on heels, feet flat, raise arms for balance.

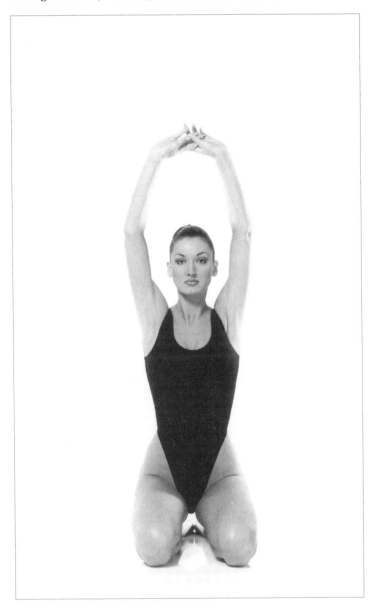

ARABIAN NIGHTS A (2)

Raise body a couple of inches.

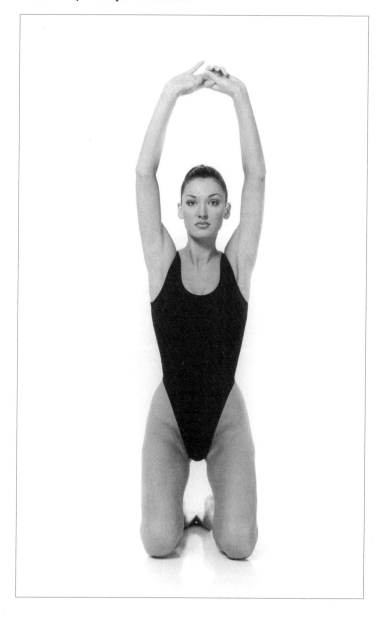

ARABIAN NIGHTS A (3)

Rotate hips up to the right, scooping pelvis upwards and pulling tummy in. Return to centre.

8 reps, repeating to the left; working thigh.

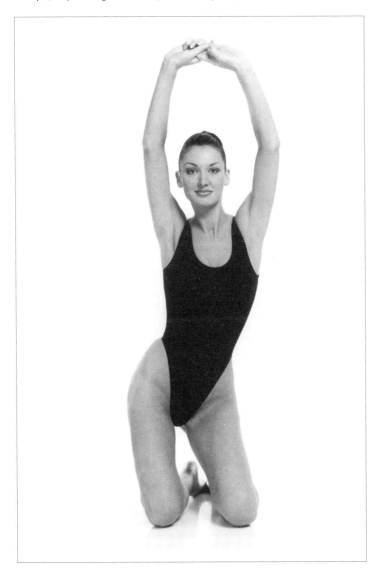

ARABIAN NIGHTS B

Combining both these exercises, rotate hips to right, back to centre, then repeat to left in figure of eight.

4 reps of sequence; working thigh.

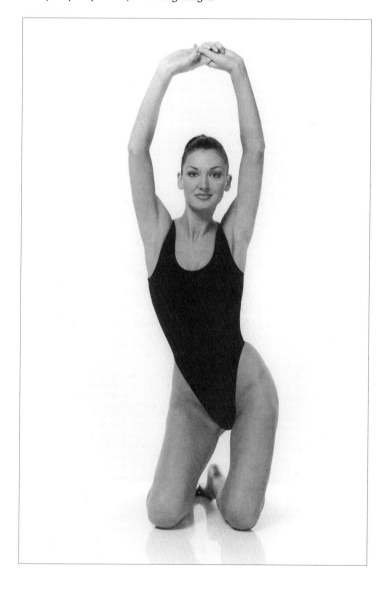

RELAXATION

When the body is tense and uptight the life-force and vital energy are shut off or misdirected. When the body is relaxed energy flows freely, helping to repair and nourish all living cells. To relax, find a place where you feel happy and comfortable and let it be your sanctuary, where you can let go of all your worries and stress. Set aside twenty or thirty minutes daily. Always allow time for relaxing after your exercises.

The best exercise I know is the corpse; they say in yoga that twenty minutes of this posture, done properly, is as beneficial as a night's sleep.

Lie on the flat of your back, head straight, palms of your hands facing upwards. Let your feet drop to left and right. Keep your head straight and point your chin into your chest. Let your mouth hang open and close your eyes. Exhale completely, taking deep breaths. Start off by relaxing your feet, then relax toes, calves, thighs, bottom, lower back, middle of back, shoulders, neck, face, forehead, eyes, mouth, chest, tummy, hands and fingers in that order. Move through your body again, letting go of all tension with each breath. Try not to think about anything; let your thoughts pass by. Stay in the stillness.

If you practise this you will find that your relaxation will gradually become more complete and contribute greatly to your wellbeing.

SUBCONSCIOUS RESHAPING

You will be on a programme of improvement. Even if it takes a bit longer, who cares? You have plenty of time. You may slip a few times or go on a binge. So what? Don't feel guilty; just start again tomorrow. One simple exercise I suggest is to get a good photograph of yourself when you looked your best. Get a few copies made. Put one on your wall, one on your fridge, one in your car, one in your wallet, and allow your mind to wander and see yourself when you were happy with your figure. This is called subconscious reshaping. If you constantly tell yourself you are fat or overweight your subconscious will oblige and programme whatever you instil in your mind. If you want to make improvements in your appearance, look at your new self instead and your subconscious will learn to accept the new image. This method is now being used in sports and personal development programmes.

If exercise is done correctly it will improve your posture; help any lower back pain; expand your oxygen capacity through correct breathing, thus giving more energy to digest food; improve your circulation and give a general sense of wellbeing.

Age is no barrier nowadays. For years it was thought that after forty the body started to deteriorate and you should take up a more gentle activity, such as knitting! There are people who exercise well into their eighties and are still making progress and improving muscle tone. Exercise helps to prevent osteoporosis by keeping the joints mobile and improving muscle strength. You can start at any age – just look at Joan Collins, Raquel Welsh, Jane Fonda. So don't let anyone convince you that you are too old to start. The feeling of wellbeing is what you were meant to have, not always being tired, irritable or stressed. Exercise can be used to treat people with depression and stress problems – with fantastic results. All you are doing is enhancing your own life-force, increasing your internal energy, giving yourself that wellbeing from the inside out.

MASSAGE

The earliest book on massage is written as far back as 3000 BC. Ki massage – which is what I recommend to my clients – was developed by the Irish Health Culture Association, which is today a leading organisation, training many therapists who go through a very strict programme to meet the standards set. With Ki massage you will experience a feeling of deep relaxation which allows you to withdraw from everyday stress and come back to face life with new energy. This has an extraordinary effect on your health and mental wellbeing and, repeated over a period of time, it brings about a very positive outlook. The goal of massage is to relax and invigorate you. It stimulates circulation in a natural way and helps to stop you getting uptight. Massage is used by doctors and osteopaths, naturpaths and healers. It is good for stiff necks, sore backs, sprains, aching feet, arthritis, depression and many other conditions. It gets the healing energy flowing in your body as a whole and it helps this energy to move to any sick or injured areas. This is particularly beneficial for the elderly or for those who are ill or incapacitated. In healthy people, massage will benefit directly the areas of sluggish circulation not affected by exercise.

A good masseur or masseuse must develop the ability to relax and become completely absorbed in the work, in order to bring about a proper state of relaxation for the client. Massage:

- Increases blood supply to the joints
- Produces muscular relaxation
- Prevents fibrosis in muscles
- Decreases the tendency to muscular atrophy
- Soothes overstimulated nerves
- Increases the value of nutrition
- Helps to remove waste more quickly

Massage also helps to remove cellulite. It can be combined with a very strict non-fat diet to cut out toxins completely, improve the circulation and help you get rid of the body fat that can cause cellulite.

Ki massage brings a sense of wellbeing that is impossible to simulate by drugs or other artificial means. You can make it part of your programme to improve your health, appearance and wellbeing.

2

WALKING

Walking is part of the programme to complement the exercises described in this book. The first point to remember is to aim for *health*, not weight loss at any cost. On the days you are not doing your floor exercises simply go for a brisk walk. Walking itself is good exercise whether you are sixteen or seventy; in fact it is one of the best exercises you can do. It strengthens the cardiovascular system, tones muscles and increases flexibility, reduces stress and burns fat. It also causes a minimum amount of stress in your body. A walker's foot receives one to one-and-a-half times the body-weight each time it strikes the ground; a runner's receives three to four times the body-weight with each stride. This means fewer injuries. Walking a mile burns the same number of calories as running a mile. Brisk walking with a moderate ten-degree incline burns more calories than jogging at the rate of five miles an hour. Fitness walking is often used by athletes as a component of an effective cross-training programme. It complements cycling, swimming and running.

Combined with a light weight-training programme and the exercises described in this book, walking could produce a new you. This is the best combination for losing fat and excess weight. Walking burns fat for energy, whereas other activities run on carbohydrate, burning short-term energy. One hour of brisk walking burns an average of 348 calories and one pound of fat equals 3,500 calories. So if you look at it this way, if you lose 348 calories for the 365 days of a year, you will have lost 127,020 calories in total: in other words, thirty-six pounds, everything else being equal, of course! Walk briskly, changing your stride every mile to avoid back or hip strain. Changing stride also helps to firm the legs and the bottom. Try walking heel-to-toe rather than shuffling your feet along. Walking correctly will help to make your journey easier and prevent shin and calf strain. If you find walking four miles an hour too hard just do two or three miles at whatever speed is right for you. Establish your own pace, make it enjoyable, find a route that is good for you. If it is convenient, try the beach or even the park, somewhere there is clean air: a high oxygen intake also helps you to burn more calories as well. Get yourself a good pair of runners or walking shoes. Don't use shoes that are ancient or hurt your feet. As you get fitter, put a little Vaseline on your heels and toes and wear good stocks to prevent friction or blisters.

For those of you who find walking too easy, stride walking may be better. Simply use light arm and ankle weights. The effect is like cross-country skiing without skiing but with the arm movements. Aim for a brisk speed of five miles an hour.

STAIR CLIMB

If you have access to a building with a lot of stairs you have at your disposal one of the best aerobic exercises of all. Climb at a pace that will not leave you exhausted for fifteen to twenty minutes for the best cardiovascular and conditioning results. Remember, walking around the kitchen or the office does not count. Happy trails!

CALORIES BURNED THROUGH DIFFERENT FORMS OF EXERCISE

	Aerobic	Effect on Muscle Tone	Calories Burned Per Hour	Special Benefits
Swimming	•••	•••	500 cals (50yds/min)	Great all-over body conditioning. Excellent for the overweight.
Tennis	•••	••	400 cals	Good cardiovascular exercise, excellent for eye-hand coordination. Enjoyable social game.
Squash	•••	••	400 cals	Excellent cardiovascular exercise. Improves reflexes.
Weight Training (non-circuit)	••	••••	700 cals	Excellent for body tone and conditioning. Great for specific problem areas.
Running	••••	•••	1,280 cals (10 mph)	Fantastic aerobic exercise, builds stamina and strength.
Cross-Country Skiing	••••	•••	700 cals	Exhilarating exercise, great for fresh air and fun. Increases lower body strength and tone.
Cycling	••••	•••	410 cals (12 mph)	A way to see the world. Great exercise for the legs. Good aerobic exercise.

3

DIET

Sometimes women who long for good, slim, shapely legs work hard but see little improvement. You have to remember that exercise on its own will never work. If you are doing thousands of leg exercises but still eating fatty worthless food nothing will happen. A lot of diets are counterproductive. They encourage dieters to count calories and starve themselves. All they eventually lose is muscle – the fat remains. Less than 5 per cent of dieters lose weight and keep it off. Starvation diets simply slow down your metabolism to help to conserve fat. What you lose is water, some fat, and muscle which is used for fuel. When you start to eat normally again you put back all the weight you lost and maybe even a little more.

The more firm muscle tissue you have, the more fat you burn off. Muscles simply need oxygen and calories and when you are on a correct low-fat diet, your fat stores, not muscle tissue, are used for fuel. You will lose that unwanted fat and firm up. Don't be discouraged by charts that show how many calories certain exercises burn off. The extra fat was probably accumulated over a long period and should be taken off slowly in the same manner. No more than two pounds a week. One pound of fat equals 3,500 calories. To lose that one pound you must eat less or do some exercise. Better again, do both.

'YO-YO' DIETING

Some people are constantly going on and off diets. A survey done in Pennslyvania State University found that people who are constantly going on and off diets eventually have a higher fat percentage. It can also be extremely bad for your heart. Your system can become very confused. You actually gain more body fat as opposed to lean muscle tone. Fooling around with different diets does not work in the long term. You will find that you gain weight and the weight you gain will be higher proportionally in fat. The Pennsylvanian State University survey also found that if you are constantly changing your diet, the weight loss from the hips and the thighs will be redistributed in the abdominal area.

It may also be possible that your system is very sluggish. The average person may be five meals behind in elimination. Often food may not be digested properly before the next meal is taken. This could be caused by a simple thing like drinking with meals. If you drink liquid with meals it may interfere with your body's hydrochloric acid, which aids digestion. The signs of food not properly digested include bad breath, strong body odour, sweating a lot, feeling tired, poor skin and lifeless hair. These problems may be aggravated by eating junk foods. To avoid these problems, try not to drink liquids with meals. Instead have liquids half an hour after your meal to give your system a chance to digest your food naturally. If you follow the diet plan contained in this book, you may think of spending just one day a week eating pears or grapes or another fruit. This would be your fast day and would help to clear out your system. It would be a good idea to go on a fast day before beginning the diet proper.

THE SECRET OF LOSING WEIGHT

If you constantly say to yourself 'I must lose weight', 'I am too fat', 'My waist is too big', it means that you are seeing yourself out of shape in the mirror. It will be very difficult for any diet to work for you because you are constantly programming your subconscious mind with negative thoughts. At the moment you are the result of what you have been thinking so you must try to change the thoughts in your mind, change your own image of yourself. If you try to change your diet without changing your mental attitude you will find yourself getting cranky, having mood swings, hunger pangs and cravings for food. If you get an incredible craving for sweets or cakes you are better off eating them because if you don't eat them with your mouth you eat them with your mind, and it is not worth getting upset over. If you break your diet, so what? Start again.

The first thing you should do is get your figure assessed, maybe in a health studio or by a friend. Look in the mirror and see how much weight you would like to lose. Find out what body type you have. Are you endomorph, mesomorph or ectomorph? Your body type will determine how slim you can expect to get. As you lie in bed, close your eyes and visualise yourself in the shape that you want to be in. If you do this last thing at night and first thing in the morning you are programming your subconscious. Repeat this in your mind, for example, the sentence, 'I will be eight stone with a figure I want' or whatever message you want to programme in. This is called mantra yoga. You will know it is working if the thought of your new figure is the first thing on your mind when you wake up in the morning. This means that your subconscious mind has accepted your programme and that it will definitely work.

But you also have to diet. Don't start a programme and eat junk food at the same time. I am totally against all starvation diets and liquid diets. If a diet is not balanced you will find that your skin and hair, your muscle tone and your whole body will suffer. For instance, if you are suffering from stress and go on a starvation diet you will certainly become more stressed. In fact, if you are stressed you need a little extra weight just to keep you stable. If you are starving yourself you become more nervous and deplete your body of vitamins, especially calcium and B-vitamins. Calcium helps to coat the nervous system and has a calming effect when taken with vitamins A and D.

If you want to go on a diet, consult someone who has experience in nutrition. The best way to lose weight is simply to visualise yourself the way you want to be, go on a good gradual diet and follow an exercise programme.

CELLULITE

There are so many products on sale to help you with weight and figure problems that it is easy to become confused or even to be misled. The prevalence of 'cottage cheese' thighs in Ireland is a boon to the cosmetic industry. Anti-cellulite creams abound, all making different claims as to how they deal with the problem. Some claim they break down cellulite to release the toxins it contains. Others claim to increase circulation to carry away the toxins that 'are the main cause of cellulite', or to release water trapped in unsightly ripples under the skin. Some go as far as to claim that their creams will remove cellulite wholesale.

Yet as Dr Peter Fodder, president of the Lipoplasty Society emphasises, there *are* no toxins, and there *is* no trapped water. Cellulite is just ordinary body fat sitting under the skin in tiny pockets separated by connective tissue. Creams or lotions cannot remove a molecule unless they contain a drug that can penetrate the skin and enter the fat underneath. All such drugs are still experimental and it will be years before the American licensing body, the Food and Drugs Administration (FDA) approves one. Then it will be strictly on prescription. That leaves changes in your lifestyle – in your diet and exercise levels in particular – as the only sure way of beating cellulite.

LOTIONS, POTIONS, DRUGS AND GADGETS

Over-the-counter weight loss remedies don't have such a good record either. Recently the FDA banned as ineffective or unhealthy more than one hundred substances that were being sold for weight control, including teas, pills and artificial sweeteners. Nor should you be tempted to use drugs to lose weight.

The majority of people who take drugs to remove body weight quickly put the weight back on. And with possible side-effects such as increased blood pressure, nausea, insomnia, permanent nervous feelings and heart palpitations – it's just not worth it!

Another alarming development of the slimming business has been to convince people that attaching machines to themselves at home and lying back to watch TV will help them lose weight. It just isn't true. At best these machines will keep the body toned. No such machines will ever burn off body fat and it is a shame that people are gullible enough to believe it.

For permanent results you have to change your lifestyle, eat a low-fat diet, exercise with light weights and aerobic exercises, cut down on tea, coffee, alcohol, sugar and junk food. Have regular massage to help to break down the waste and fat that has accumulated over a long period. It may take a while to achieve the desired results, but see your progress as a long-term project. Allow yourself one year to reinvent yourself with your new figure or physique.

Remember, if you have a lot of fat on your tummy, hips or legs, the only real way of reducing the fat is to stop eating it. Fat builds fat.

Always avoid all low-calorie diets, starvation diets and liquid diets. They will never yield permanent results.

YOUR DIETARY PLAN

This diet is designed to help you lose unwanted body fat, attain a firmer figure and also increase your energy. It is a diet moderately high in proteins and carbohydrates, cutting fat and added sugar to a minimum. Protein helps the body to firm up and carbohydrates supply the energy. This is not a fad diet and it should form the basis of a new healthier eating pattern. The main constituents are: fruit, vegetables (raw or cooked), grains, beans, skimmed milk, along with low-fat and fat-free protein.

Before we look at a seven-day menu plan the following lists will help you to choose the best foods for your diet.

LOW/NON-FAT CARBOHYDRATES
Bread
Rice
Potatoes
Cooked Vegetables
Raw Salads
Bananas
Dried Fruit
Beans
Sprouts
Pasta
Noodles

FRUIT
All fruit except avocados and olives are very low in fat.

LOW/FAT- FREE PROTEINS
Round steak/mince
Liver, kidneys
Chicken or turkey without skin
White fish
(Oily fish such as salmon mackerel, herring or sardines could

be taken once a week)
Shellfish
Tuna
Cottage cheese
Skim milk
Eggs (free-range)
(The whites are fat-free, the yolks are fat. Omelettes or scrambled eggs can be made using three whites to one yolk.)
TVP (textured vegetable protein), a soya meat substitute

DRINKS

- Most peple do not drink enough water. Try to take two pints a day (non-sparkling) either between or after meals.
- Fizzy drinks and many carton fruit juices have added sugar and should be avoided.
- Two glasses of wine a week is allowed. Beer, however, is not desirable because it has a bloating effect.
- Cocoa made with skim milk is fine.
- Herbal teas are preferable to tea or coffee.
- Fruit juices are fine if they are sugar-free.

FOODS TO AVOID

Butter, margarine, low-fat spreads, pastry, cakes, desserts, biscuits, jams, oil, fried food, cream, ice-cream, mayonnaise, whole milk (try to use skim milk only), salad dressing, cheese and yogurt unless fat-free, all pork products and fatty meats, avocados, olives, nuts, all fizzy soft drinks, sugar, all junk foods/fast foods.

SNACKS

- Piece of fruit
- Vegetable sticks, such as carrots and celery
- Dried fruit in small amounts: raisins, figs, apricots
- Popcorn

Personal Notes

MENUS

(Please refer to the recipe section for the dishes marked *)

DAY 1

BREAKFAST
Orange juice
1 boiled egg
$^1/_2$ slice of toast and scraping of butter
Tea or coffee (no sugar – use sweetener)

LUNCH
4 ozs cottage cheese
Pineapple salad
2 crispbreads

DINNER
Roast chicken (no skin) or chicken provençale*
Rice
Courgette
Baked apple with cinnamon and raisins

DAY 2

BREAKFAST
Porridge, cooked with raisins and skimmed milk
Tea or coffee

LUNCH
Turkey breast and salad sandwich

DINNER
White fish*
2 small potatoes
Green beans
Natural yogurt and honey

DAY 3

BREAKFAST
Milk shake – skim milk blended with banana and honey or maple syrup
$1/2$ slice of toast and sugar-free jam

LUNCH
Mushroom omelette
1 pear

DINNER
Vegetable stir-fry and rice
Pineapple

DAY 4

BREAKFAST
$1/2$ pink grapefruit
1 rasher – grilled
$1/2$ slice of toast and scraping of butter

LUNCH
Tuna salad in pitta bread
Slice of melon

DINNER
Lasagne or bolognaise* or vegetable casserole*
Fat-free cheesecake

DAY 5

BREAKFAST
Apple juice
Scrambled eggs
$^1/_2$ slice of toast
Tea or coffee

LUNCH
Toasted cheese sandwich
Fromage frais and fruit

DINNER
Grilled mackerel and seed mustard
Spinach
Boiled potatoes
Sorbet or summer pudding

DAY 6

BREAKFAST
Shredded wheat and sliced banana with skim milk
Toasted muffin and honey
Tea or coffee

LUNCH
Vegetable soup
Baked potato with cottage cheese
Tangerines

DINNER
Stuffed pepper with minced lamb
Boiled rice
Strawberries

DAY 7

BREAKFAST
Fresh mango or papaya or melon
Pancakes and maple syrup
Tea or coffee

LUNCH
Prawns and avocado salad
Wholegrain crackers
1 peach

DINNER
Roast pork steak stuffed with apple
Broccoli
Mashed potato
Rhubarb snow*

RECIPES

FISH

BAKED SOLE/PLAICE (SERVES 1)

6 ozs black sole
juice of $^1/_2$ lemon
'Fry Light' sunflower or olive oil cooking spray
Garlic powder (optional)
Black pepper

Place sole on tinfoil. Spray with Fry Light and pour lemon juice over fish. Sprinkle on garlic and black pepper. Fold over tinfoil, tightly sealing edges, so that none of the juices escape. Bake in a moderate oven, 350°F, gas mark 4, for 25 minutes.

CURRIED ANGLER (SERVES 1)

6 ozs angler fish
$1/2$ small onion, finely diced
1 level tsp curry powder
$2/3$ cup boiled water
3 tbls apricot juice (unsweetened)
$1/2$ apricot

Dissolve curry powder in boiled water. Simmer onion in $1/2$ of the curry juice until soft. Add fish, cut in small pieces, with remainder of curry juice. Cook gently for 5 minutes. Then add apricot juice and $1/2$ apricot. Cover and simmer for 20 minutes. Serve on a bed of finely chopped spinach.

ORANGE-FLAVOURED COD (SERVES 1)

6 ozs cod
Juice of 1 orange
Salt
Black pepper
Sprig parsley

Steam cod until soft. Put orange juice, salt and pepper into frying pan. Bring nearly to the boil, add cod, skin removed, and simmer for 5 minutes. Decorate with parsley and serve hot or cold.

BAKED COD (SERVES 1)

6 ozs cod
1 hard-boiled egg
Juice of $1/2$ fresh grapefruit
5 ozs natural yogurt
Black pepper

Place fish in a casserole dish. In a separate bowl mix yogurt, black pepper and grapefruit juice. Finely grate the hard-boiled egg and mix into sauce. Pour over fish, cover and bake in a moderate oven, 350°F, gas mark 4, for 30 minutes.

WHITING IN YOGURT (SERVES 1)

6 ozs whiting
1/4 lb mushrooms
5 ozs natural yogurt
Fines herbes
Black pepper

Place whiting (skin removed) in a casserole dish. Add mushrooms, (peel only if necessary), pour over yogurt and sprinkle with herbs and black pepper. Cover and bake in moderate oven, 350°F, gas mark 4, for 25 minutes.

MEAT

VEAL CASSEROLE (SERVES 4)

1 1/2 lbs stewing veal
3 tbls tomato purée
5 ozs natural yogurt
1 medium onion (peeled and chopped)
Paprika
Black pepper
1/2 chicken stock cube
1/4 pint water

Chop meat into cubes. Blend tomato purée with yogurt. Add chopped onion, paprika and black pepper. Dissolve stock cube in water. Place meat in a casserole dish and cover with stock. Then pour over the yogurt, mix and cover with tinfoil. Cook in a pre-heated oven, 375°F, gas mark 4, and reduce temperature to 325°F, gas mark 3, after 5 minutes for a further 45 minutes.

HAMBURGER (SERVES 1)

6 ozs very lean mince
$1/2$ small onion, finely chopped
1 stick celery (finely chopped)
Sprig parsley
Garlic powder (optional)
Tarragon
Black pepper
$1/2$ egg (beaten)

Put mince in a bowl. Add onion, celery, parsley, pinch of garlic powder, tarragon and black pepper. Mix all ingredients well together. Form into hamburger shape with palm of hands and dip in beaten egg, coating well all sides. Place under a moderate grill and cook, making sure to grill both sides. Approximately 4 minutes each side (rare), 6 minutes each side (well done).

CHICKEN PROVENÇALE (SERVES 1)

$1/2$ green pepper
$1/2$ red pepper
1 small onion
4 ozs mushrooms
1 clove garlic, crushed
14 ozs canned peeled tomatoes
2 tbls tomato purée
1 breast of chicken (skin removed)
Herbs (rosemary and thyme)
Black pepper

Cut peppers into strips, chop onion and clean mushrooms. Put onion, peppers, garlic in a saucepan with tomatoes and half the tomato purée. Cook gently for 5 minutes, then add chicken, mushrooms, herbs and pepper. Bring to the boil and simmer gently for 15 minutes. Add remainder of tomato purée and cook for a further 20 minutes.

BOLOGNAISE (SERVES 1)

1 small onion
1/2 green pepper
3 ozs mushrooms
1 clove garlic (crushed)
31/2 ozs tomato purée
11/2 cups water
6 ozs very lean mince meat
Black pepper
Salt

Put chopped onion, green pepper cut into strips, mushrooms cut in quarters and crushed garlic clove in a saucepan with the tomato purée dissolved in $1^1/_2$ cups water. Bring to the boil and simmer for 5 minutes. Then add mince meat, black pepper and a pinch of salt and cook gently for 20 minutes.

PORK TENDERLOIN WITH ROASTED APPLES AND PEARS (SERVES 4)

1 oz plain flour
1 tsp sage-and-apple seasoning (or use dried mixed herbs)
Salt and pepper
15 ozs pork tenderloin
2 medium apples
2 medium pears
1 tbl lemon juice

Preheat oven to 400°F, gas mark 6. Sprinkle the flour, sage-and-apple seasoning or mixed herbs, salt and pepper on to a plate. Mix well. Rinse the pork fillet, but do not pat dry. Slice thickly, then coat the pieces in the seasoned flour. Arrange on a rack positioned over a roasting tin. Quarter and core the apples and pears, without peeling them. Sprinkle with lemon juice and place next to the pork. Roast for 30–35 minutes, until the pork is cooked and the fruit is tender.

VEGETABLES/SALADS

WINTER VEGETABLE CASSEROLE (SERVES 4)

1 tbl olive or vegetable oil
1 clove garlic (crushed)
2 onions (chopped)
2 celery sticks (chopped)
8 ozs swede or turnip (chopped)
2 carrots (sliced)
6 ozs cauliflower or broccoli (broken into florets)
8 ozs button mushrooms
14 oz can chopped tomatoes
1 oz red lentils
1 oz pearl barley
1 tbl paprika
$^1/_2$ pint vegetable stock
1 tbl fresh parsley (chopped)
2 tbls cornflour, blended with a little water
Salt and pepper

Preheat the oven to 350°F, gas mark 4. Heat the oil in a flameproof casserole dish and sauté the garlic and onions for 3-4 minutes. Then add the celery, swede or turnip, carrots and cauliflower or broccoli. Cook, stirring, for 2-3 more minutes. Add the mushrooms, tomatoes, lentils, pearl barley and paprika, stirring well, then add the stock and parsley. Bring to the boil, then cover and transfer to oven. Bake for 40-45 minutes. Remove the casserole from the oven, stir in the blended cornflour and season. Bake for 5 more minutes.

CARROT PURÉE (SERVES 4–5)

2 lbs carrots
1 small onion
Garlic powder (optional)
Black pepper
Chives

Dice carrots, slice onion and put in saucepan with just enough water to cover. Bring to the boil and cook gently until almost soft. Allow to cool then put into blender and blend until a thick purée is achieved. Put back into saucepan and add garlic powder, black pepper and chives to taste, mixing well. Serve hot or cold.

For a variation in flavour, tomatoes, turnips or *fines herbes* may be added to the purée.

SALADE NIÇOISE FOR SLIMMERS (SERVES 4)

1 head cos lettuce
8 ozs green beans (lightly cooked)
1 green pepper
1 red pepper
2 hard-boiled eggs
4 tomatoes (chopped)
1 cup chinese leaves (unshredded)
10 pitted black olives
8 anchovies (well drained)

(To drain anchovies put them in a small bowl of milk for 2 hours and strain)

Arrange lettuce around the salad bowl. Chop the hard-boiled eggs in a separate bowl. Add french beans, red and green peppers (cut in rings), chopped tomatoes, olives, shredded chinese leaves and anchovies. Mix well with a vinaigrette dressing and add to salad bowl.

RATATOUILLE (SERVES 3-4)

1 medium onion
1 green pepper
1 red pepper
2 cloves garlic, crushed
14 oz can whole tomatoes
2 ozs tomato purée
$1/4$ lb mushrooms
1 medium aubergine
Herbs (rosemary and thyme)
Pinch of salt
Black pepper
2 courgettes

Slice onion in rings. Cut green and red peppers in strips and crush garlic. Pour half the tomatoes (7 ozs) into a saucepan and add the onion, peppers in strips, and garlic. Bring to the boil and simmer for 5 minutes. Add the rest of the tomatoes, tomato purée, mushrooms (whole), aubergine (cut into thick rings), herbs, salt and black pepper. Cook gently for 15 minutes, adding more seasoning to taste if necessary. Add the courgette, washed but not peeled and cut into thick slices. Continue to cook for a further 10 minutes. If the liquid becomes too scarce, add water or tomato juice accordingly. Serve hot or cold.

SPINACH SALAD (SERVES 2-3)

$1^1/2$ lbs fresh spinach
$1/2$ medium onion (finely sliced)
2 hard-boiled eggs
Black pepper
Vinaigrette dressing

Clean and chop spinach, discarding stalks. Mix with sliced onion. Pour 3 tbls vinaigrette dressing over salad and arrange sliced eggs on top. Leave to soften for 1 hour before eating. Yogurt dressing may be substituted if desired.

COLESLAW (SERVES 2)

2 cups grated carrots
3 cups shredded white cabbage
1/2 cup grated onion
Black pepper
Vinaigrette/yogurt dressing

Mix carrots, cabbage and onion in a salad bowl. Sprinkle over black pepper and mix well with 2 tbls vinaigrette or yogurt dressing.

WALDORF SALAD (SERVES 3)

3 cups celery (finely diced)
1 green apple (hard)
1 small onion
1/2 cup chopped walnuts
Black pepper

Cut apple in quarters and finely slice. Grate the onion and add to the finely diced celery and apple. Add walnuts and mix all ingredients well together with 3 tbls yogurt dressing. Sprinkle black pepper over salad.

(If salad is not to be eaten immediately, soak apple in lemon juice to prevent it from turning brown.)

TURKISH SALAD (SERVES 3)

1/4 lb mushrooms
1/2 cucumber
Yogurt dressing
Black pepper

Clean mushrooms and slice finely. Peel and dice cucumber. Mix together with dressing. Sprinkle over with black pepper. Leave to soften 2-3 hours before eating.

FRENCH BEANS À LA MENTHE (SERVES 3-4)

1 lb french beans
2 tsp low-fat spread
2 tsp dried mint
Black pepper

Lightly boil the french beans until almost soft. Drain. Add low-fat spread, mint and black pepper, mixing well. Serve hot or cold.

PEPPER AND CUCUMBER SALAD (SERVES 1-2)

$^1/_2$ cucumber
$^1/_2$ green pepper
$^1/_2$ red pepper
Black pepper
2 tbls vinaigrette dressing

Slice cucumber and cut in quarters. Slice peppers in thin strips and dice. Mix peppers and cucumber in a salad bowl, sprinkle with black pepper and mix well with 2 tbls vinaigrette dressing.

TOMATO AND CUCUMBER SALAD (SERVES 2)

3 tomatoes
$^1/_2$ cucumber
1 small onion
1 tbl vinaigrette dressing
Fines herbes
Black pepper

Finely dice onion. Slice tomatoes in rings and slice cucumber finely. Mix in a bowl. Pour 1 tbl vinaigrette dressing over salad and sprinkle with herbs and black pepper.

TOMATOES VINAIGRETTE (SERVES 1)

2 tomatoes, sliced
2 tsp finely sliced onion
Fines herbes
Black pepper
1 tbl vinaigrette dressing

Mix all ingredients together in a bowl and pour 1 tbl vinaigrette over salad.

CHICORY SALAD (SERVES 2)

6 ozs chicory
4 ozs low-fat cottage cheese
10 walnuts (finely chopped)
10 radishes (sliced)
vinaigrette or yogurt dressing

Chop chicory. Finely slice radishes. Mix all the ingredients together with a vinaigrette or yogurt dressing.

SALAD DRESSINGS

YOGURT DRESSING

4 ozs natural yogurt
1 tsp mustard powder
1 tsp dried mint (optional)
$1/2$ tsp garlic powder (optional)
1 tbl lemon juice
Black pepper

Shake all ingredients in a screwtop jar and chill. For variation in flavour, 2 tsp tomato purée or $1/2$ tsp curry powder may be added to the dressing.

VINAIGRETTE

2 tbls oil (sunflower or olive)
3 tbls wine vinegar or fresh lemon juice
1 tsp mustard
1/2 clove garlic, crushed (optional)
Fines herbes
Black pepper

Put all ingredients in a screwtop jar and shake well. If using garlic, allow the dressing to stand for 1-2 hours before serving to strengthen the garlic flavour.

DESSERTS

RHUBARB SNOW (SERVES 2)

1 lb fresh rhubarb
3 teaspoons fructose
1/2 tsp ground ginger
2 egg whites

Stew rhubarb, fructose and ginger with just enough water to cover. Beat egg whites until stiff, then fold egg whites into rhubarb and mix. Place under a hot grill until egg whites become golden. Serve hot.

GOOSEBERRY FOOL (SERVES 4)

1 lb fresh gooseberries
3 teaspoons fructose
4 ozs natural yogurt

Stew gooseberries and fructose with just enough water to cover. When cooked, allow to cool. Then add yogurt. Blend and chill.

CALORIE CHART

(This chart is given for reference only. We do not recommend that you follow a strict low-calorie diet or become an obsessive calorie counter.)

	Portion	Calories
BEVERAGES		
Beer	8 oz	101
Coffee	8 oz	2
Cola drink	8 oz	88
Dry wine	8 oz	204
Martini	3.5 oz	140
Skim milk	8 oz	89
Whole milk	8 oz	159
BREAD AND CEREALS		
Bran flakes 40%	1 cup (40 gm)	143
Cornflakes	1 cup (25 gm)	98
Oatmeal, cooked	1 cup (236 gm)	130
Rye	1 slice (23 gm)	56
Whole wheat	1 slice (23 gm)	55
CONDIMENTS AND SAUCES		
Cider vinegar	1 tb (15 gm)	3
French dressing	1 tb (15 gm)	62
Hollandaise	1 tb (21 gm)	48
Italian dressing	1 tb (15 gm)	83
Mayonnaise	1 tb (14 gm)	101
Mustard	1 tb (12 gm)	11
Soy sauce	1 tb (15 gm)	8
Tomato ketchup	1 tb (17 gm)	19
CREAM		
Half & Half	1 tb (15 gm)	20
Whipping	1 cup (8 oz)	860

DAIRY PRODUCTS

Cheddar cheese	1 oz	112
Cottage cheese	1 cup (8 oz)	235
Cream cheese	1 tb (14 gm)	53
Gruyère cheese	1 oz	115

DESSERTS

Apple pie	1 piece (135 gm)	346
Brownies	1 slice (50 gm)	243
Cake doughnuts	1 med	33
Chocolate chip cookies	1 med (9 gm)	46
Devil's food cake, no icing	1 slice (45 gm)	165
Ice-cream, all flavours	1 cup	389
Peanut cookie	1 large (14 gm)	66
Pumpkin pie	1 piece (130 gm)	274
Sugar	1 tb (12 gm)	46

EGGS

Boiled, poached or raw	1 med	79
Fried	1 med	108

FATS AND OILS

Butter	1 tb (14 gm)	100
Safflower oil	1 tb (14 gm)	124

FISH AND SEAFOODS

Whiting, baked or poached	1 lb (454 gm)	720
Cod, poached	1 lb (454 gm)	740
Crabmeat	1 lb (454 gm)	398
Lobster, steamed	1 med (200 gm)	179
Oysters, raw	1 cup (240 gm)	152
Salmon, poached	1 lb (454 gm)	824

FRUITS AND JUICES

Apple	1 med (130 gm)	76
Avocado	1 large (216 gm)	361
Banana	1 med (150 gm)	128
Blueberries	1 cup (140 gm)	87
Cantaloupe melon	1 quarter (100 gm)	30
Dried dates	1 med (10 gm)	27
Dried figs	1 med (38 gm)	30
Grapefruit	1 med (260 gm)	108
Lemon juice	1 tb (15 gm)	4
Ripe olives	1 large (7 gm)	13
Papaya	1 large (400 gm)	156
Peach	1 med (114 gm)	43
Pear	1 med (182 gm)	111
Raisins	1 cup (160 gm)	462
Raspberries	1 cup (133 gm)	76
Strawberries	1 cup (149 gm)	55

GRAINS

Brown rice, raw	1 cup (190 gm)	744
Wheat bran	1 oz (29 gm)	62
Wheat germ	1 tb (6 gm)	24
White rice, raw	1 cup (191 gm)	675

MEAT, POULTRY AND GAME

Beef round steak, lean	1 lb (454 gm)	856
Chicken, steamed, no skin	1 lb (454 gm)	616
Ham	1 lb (454 gm)	1309
Hamburger, reg. cooked	4 oz (100 gm)	188
Lamb leg, roasted	1 lb (454 gm)	1264
Pork roast	1 lb (454 gm)	1690
Sirloin, T-bone, porterhouse	1 lb (454 gm)	1848
Turkey, white meat	1 lb (454 gm)	797

NUTS

Almonds, dried	1 cup (140 gm)	765
Cashews, unsalted	1 cup (100 gm)	569
Peanut butter	1 tb (15 gm)	88
Roasted peanuts	1 cup (240 gm)	1418
Sesame seeds	1 cup (230 gm)	1339

VEGETABLES

Artichoke	1 small (100 gm)	44
Asparagus	1 spear (16 gm)	3.2
Baked potato	1 med (100 gm)	93
Beansprouts	1 cup (50 gm)	18
Broccoli	1 cup (150 gm)	39
Carrot, raw	1 large (100 gm)	42
Cauliflower, raw	1 cup (100 gm)	27
Celery stalk, raw	1 large (50 gm)	8
Corn, whole kernel	1 cup (200 gm)	132
Cucumber	$^1/_2$ med (50 gm)	8
Green beans, cooked	1 cup (125 gm)	31
Green onions	1 bulb (8 gm)	4
Green pepper	1 large (100 gm)	22
Iceberg lettuce	3.5 oz (100 gm)	13
Lima beans, cooked	1 cup (195 gm)	265
Spinach, steamed	1 cup (100 gm)	23
Tomato, raw	1 med (150 gm)	33

4

SHOULD I CONSULT A DOCTOR
BEFORE EXERCISING?

If you are a first-time exerciser doctors recommend the following guidelines before starting a programme. If you are thirty or older and need to exercise it is a good idea to consult your doctor. Write out your exercise programme and show it to your doctor for his opinion. If you are under thirty and have any reason to suspect that you may have heart trouble, blood pressure problems, breathlessness, bone or joint problems or any old injury, or any medical condition that might need special attention in an exercise programme – such as diabetes – consult your doctor. If you are confident that none of these items affect you, you can start on a sensible gradual programme that is tailored to your needs.

DOS AND DON'TS

- Don't do high-impact aerobics.
- Don't overdo step aerobics classes as they build up the calves.
- Avoid very high-heeled shoes as they make the calf develop higher up the leg.
- Jogging or too much running can build up the outside of

the thighs.

- Avoid heavy squats with weights, especially flat squats – they develop the bottom.
- Walk an average of four miles in one hour.
- Change your walking stride every mile to avoid hip strain.
- Find a block of offices that has stairs and run up three to four flights of stairs quickly – good for the bottom.
- Do a good stretching programme.
- Remember that 70 per cent of success is down to diet, genetics and God.

MEASUREMENTS (6-WEEK CHART)

Week	1	2	3	4	5	6
Height						
Weight						
Neck						
Bicep						
Chest/Bust						
Waist						
Hips						
Thigh						
Calf						

INDEX OF RECIPES

LIST OF STRETCHES AND EXERCISES